DOCTORS
&
MEDICINE

HENRI MONDOR

OF THE « ACADÉMIE FRANÇAISE »

DOCTORS & MEDICINE

in the works of

DAUMIER

NOTES AND CATALOGUE BY

JEAN ADHÉMAR

Assistant-Director of the « Cabinet des Estampes »

PREFACE BY

ARTHUR W. HEINTZELMAN

Keeper of Prints, Boston Public Library

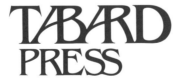

TABARD
PRESS

Tabard Press
156 Fifth Avenue
New York, N.Y. 10010

ISBN: 0-914427-23-7

Printed and bound in the United States of America

A FEW general comments on the theme and composition of Doctors and Medicine *will be helpful to better understand this book and the work of Honoré Daumier. The reader can turn these pages, print by print, to appraise the running annotations and captions and literary meaning of each subject; or, he can study the lithographs individually for artistic appreciation and enjoyment. By bringing together this selection of satirical and analytical illustrations that concentrate on the practice, and practitioner, in medicine, a new interest is created in Daumier's œuvre for the manners and habits of today resemble, in many ways, those of Daumier's time.*

Daumier had the power to grasp life in terms of its eternal and unchanging verities. His style and humor can never be confused with the work of another; yet, there is something more. Almost miraculously his pictorial records of the middle of the nineteenth century, are with little variation, very close in spirit to the twentieth. Human emotions, family problems and amusing situations are familiar. This is forcibly and candidly illustrated in the prints of medical subjects and medical expressions selected from the vast representation of rich impressions of Daumier's lithographs in the collection at the Bibliothèque Nationale in Paris.

Prominent among the illustrations we find a number of subjects from Daumier's celebrated series of «Robert Macaire». He drew this character from the hero of a melodrama, L'Auberge des Adrets, *which, at the time, was revived by the well-known French actor, Frédérick Lemaître, and Daumier used him as a model for a number of his ideas and opinions. We are told by Thackeray that the play was a witless performance with an extravagant style of conversation, exaggerated sentiments, social and political actions which would typify a villain. Daumier has created Macaire as a person of consequence in numerous professions befitting this volume : a doctor, pharmacist and patient; and he is a character who reflects questionable impersonations as a knave, a quack and a humbug.*

Being the son of a glazier and an amateur poet, Daumier knew what it meant to be a member of the poverty-stricken lower class. All through the work of this artist there is ample evidence that he abhorred everything in government or in the social structure that deprived a man of his individuality. For years he worked with Charles Philipon, editor of la Caricature and le Charivari, both radical journals which championed the common individualist against the crushing force of moneyed interests represented by the snobbish and self-satisfied middle class. Daumier's love of freedom can readily be seen in the pages of this book. His state of mind can be interpreted as the spirit of the age, for he lived in a period which was laying the groundwork for democracy in France, and his great talent made its contribution to the national upheaval.

His vast œuvre in lithography gives us a panorama of France under Louis-Philippe, the Second Empire, and the ideas expressed in his lithographs possess three driving forces : romanticism, individuality and freedom. While poking fun at the past, especially classic drama and the worn-out traditions of the nobility, he was intensely interested in self expression, personal emotions and human worth. There is nothing sentimental in Daumier, and his humor always defended the little man, the citizen and the workman.

It is obvious that nothing escaped Daumier's crayon. The very plan of this book, which features episodes in the subject of medicine, is an interesting record of his wide range of ideas in which his quick-pointed humor takes us into amusing and sometimes near-dramatic situations. These cartoons, which are works of art, are in reality lessons that made people think. Even today, these lithographs have the power of shaking us out of our complacency, old-fashioned ideas and moralisms.

In examining these illustrations, we get the impression that Daumier found the full range of his talent and interpretive perfection in all the possibilities of lithography. So directly and simply is the story told and executed, that the meaning and bare foundation of his art cannot help but give full interest to this unique book. The subjects are homely, if you will, but emphasize his compositions which are conceived with the desire to find an answer to a crying need, or to reveal a problem which burdened his time and people.

Daumier's lithographs which were selected for this publication are subtle, yet they appeal with such direct understanding of his subject that they require little artistic insight and comprehension. To the untrained eye the message is not overshadowed by the depth of Daumier's art and the simplicity of his intention to expose or remedy. Our imaginations are stimulated by experiences and situations similar to those of which we have been victims or beneficiaries. Men, women and children in need of medical assistance tell the story in this narrative which can be told and interpreted over and over again, and for this reason it deserves to be classified as modern for all time. Daumier's work remains contemporary, for through these great prints that possess the eager, dauntless and insatiable spirit of life, he proves he is a universal and timeless master.

ARTHUR W. HEINTZELMAN

Keeper of Prints, Boston Public Library

THIS selection of Daumier's lithographs on the subject of the medical profession is based on an idea that is at once natural and original. So far, they have never been presented in a separate collection except by G. Beytout and L. Sergent, and that was many years ago.

Historians of art and social customs have rarely isolated this section of a life-work that is multiple, unconventional and often inspired, but unbelievably and discouragingly prolific. Daumier's four thousand lithographic prints, his innumerable drawings, the countless notes made in his studio, are generally classified according to his major themes : the legal profession, the bourgeoisie, parliament, the humiliated and insulted lower classes — not to mention the Church, the financial world and the police, for whom Daumier, who was as good-hearted as he was ferocious, had little liking. Yet it was inevitable that he should have reserved a goodly part of his observation and satirical wit for the medical profession. Over a hundred plates, numerous drawings and a few paintings testify to these incursions, for which a number of reasons can be specified or imagined.

First of all, it is in accordance with the oldest literary traditions that doctors should be involved in the endless charges brought by malcontents against established institutions, by the frivolous-minded against everything serious, by writers against science, by the ignorant against any subjects they find hard to understand, and finally by the sick or born grumblers against the men who heal them slowly or incompletely, or who appear to tend them roughly and automatically rather than with sympathy. These have been subjects of discord since time immemorial.

If the medical profession were able to attain to all its own goals, or simply to keep all its promises; if doctors were all infallible and personally irreproach-

7

able, their methods perfect and their disinterestedness obvious — then medical science would be a sacred, an almost holy thing, and writers and artists would be deprived of a fine subject on which to exercise their talents. But medical science, thank goodness, is still human and temporal. Those who practise it have always considered satires on their profession relevant, and indeed useful, but have put up with them less for such considerations than for their own pleasure. There is nothing masochistic in their applause of Molière and they have proved their forgiveness by giving a banquet in honor of the author of *Knock*[1]. Daumier's caricatures, whether they are subtle, cruel or fantastic, invariably move or amuse them.

Was the medical profession as depicted by this great visionary larger than life or colored by his own romanticism? No doubt it is simply an effect of art that makes it appear so. Ever since Balzac, there have been Balzacian lawyers and clients; since Zola and Maupassant there have been peasants such as they imagined and it has been said that shadows have been blue since the time of the Impressionists. It is true that our modern doctors can hardly recognize themselves in these stylized and caricatured ancestors. Nor, doubtless, did the doctors of a century ago consider these portraits lifelike — as we shall see, they cut better figures than this. Perhaps Daumier helped them to correct certain failings. The motto *castigat ridendo mores* (that a poet composed for a harlequin's backcloth and that has since become a proverb) can be applied to all professions and all social classes. Mankind feels the need of a deforming mirror so that it may laugh at its own image encountered at some street corner, in a magazine or at the circus.

Honoré Daumier was one of these fundamentally discontented men. He was a natural non-conformist, always in opposition, who was able to cast off scruples, timidity and prudence through the fall of the old régime and the advent of a considerable measure of political instability. Such reformers, whether they were motivated by hatred or, like Daumier, by generosity, had existed for centuries. We hear of them in the Middle Ages and even among the Gauls, but they were generally to be found among the well-to-do and the privileged, and they had contented themselves with champing at their gilded bits. Guy Patin taught at the «Collège de France», Saint-Évremond was a high-ranking officer, Voltaire a big landowner and, as we should say today, a capitalist. With the coming of the nineteenth century, the Third Estate raised its voice.

8

Strangely enough, the best critics of the Bourgeoisie were its own members, as if the malcontents in question could not forgive some of their peers for having attained leading positions in the country. They could never find enough cruel and sarcastic things to say about the new dignitaries, sons of the Revolution who had become conservatives and whom they accused of being profiteers on the material plane and philistines on the spiritual.

Daumier played an active part in the revolution that was in continual foment against the Bourgeoisie and its allies. All his contemporaries were aware of this and Michelet wrote him a pompous letter in which he declared : « Through you the people will be enabled to speak to the people! » Jacques Arago, brother of the famous scientist, called him « the Paul-Louis Courier of lithography[2] ». Nothing could have described him better. Though he had never been in the Artillery, never became a humanist and never had to suffer from the infidelities of his wife, this ardent son of Marseilles greatly resembled the vine-grower of the domain of «La Chavonnière». He had much in common with Béranger too. The latter was not the genius that some of the best minds of his time believed him to be but his voice was eloquent in favor of an ideology that we should describe today as of the Left, and on which a large proportion of Frenchmen were reared between 1815 and 1900. We can only form a reasonable judgement of it by imagining ourselves back in the moral rather than the political climate of this three-quarters of a century. The men who followed in the steps of the free-thinkers of the seventeenth century and the philosophers of the eighteenth, had attained freedom at last, even when they were repressed and persecuted by the authorities. They had an immense public following and neither they nor their adversaries — whom this outlook threw into rage and despair — could doubt that they would gradually win the day. When Daumier attacked doctors, he was thus attacking one of the flanks of the opposing army. According to him, they were all profiteers, mouthers of garrulous clichés and mountebanks. He does not seem to have heard of the work of such men as Pinel, Bichat, Laënnec, Dupuytren, Bouillaud and so many others. Indeed, if his engravings were to be rediscovered by an archeologist after some cataclysm, there would be nothing in them to reveal that the artist was an actual contemporary of Claude Bernard.

There can be no question of attacking the general ideas of a man whose function was to make people smile or laugh, or at the most, to stir up ironic indignation in the least complacent. One might as well reproach Gustave Flaubert for having invented Bouvard and Pécuchet at the very period when a beneficent industrialization and serious scholarship were just being born or hold it against Henri Monnier[3] that he created Monsieur Prudhomme at a time when the world was being transformed by the inventions of Jacquard, Seguin and Lenoir, who were all members of the Bourgeoisie.

Caricaturists, like novelists, generally see only the pathetic or grotesque side of people in all circumstances. As for technical progress in whatever sphere, they are, or appear to be, indifferent to it. Thus Honoré Daumier was chiefly struck by those aspects of politicians, magistrates, business men and doctors that appealed to his mood and to a good heart that he rather enjoyed displaying in public. Baudelaire once paid him a tribute in which he remarked that Daumier was acquainted with all the human monsters, the terrifying, sinister or grotesque characters that can be found in any great city and in modern society. Perhaps both the poet and the artist were inclined to believe that the end of the world was drawing near. But just as Rome survived long after Martial, Juvenal, Tacitus and others had painted what they believed to be its death agonies, so the nineteenth century, depicted as stupid and absurd by its sons and grandsons, appears to some of us now in a far better light.

A revolution was beginning within the ranks of the medical profession itself and under the very eyes of its detractors. Certain necessary changes in the behavior of doctors may have been hastened by witty or spiteful criticism, but these changes were due to the important scientific discoveries made at this time. Once these men knew more about the reasons for disease and its treatment, they soon became simpler in their manner and language, less pompous and arrogant than their predecessors.

Daumier's criticisms were never gratuitous or merely aggressive. Like many humorous writers, he was of a melancholy disposition and, like many tormented spirits, kindly, with the result that his sensibility manifested itself in rather naïve reactions to the workings of an imperfect world. His energetic depiction of *le Mal et sa Séquelle* proves what Baudelaire has called «la beauté de son cœur», but virtue rarely inspires good poetry and the verses dedicated to him by the poet are for once almost execrable. Artists and writers who set out to represent reality in its ugliest, most vulgar and most unworthy aspects are doubtless idealists but they are also often hypersensitive. There was also the risk that the blackness of thousands of such lithographs might eventually darken the painters' palette. However, we may well feel even greater distrust of artists who find everything in human nature good, and can see nothing wrong in the coarsest pleasures or in those who enjoy them.

As for Daumier, he followed a contrary tradition that was of relatively recent origin — that of Callot and Hogarth, who were acutely conscious of the horror and misery in the lives of the vagrants they depicted.   It is curious, by the way, that the descendant of this Lorrainer and this Englishman should have been a man of Provence.   There was, however, little of Mediterranean gaiety in Honoré Daumier, contemporary and compatriot of the jovial Joseph Méry[4]. He is one of the many examples that prove the falseness of the rather childish idea that all Southerners are frivolous.   Indeed, he can best be compared to a man who came from even farther South than himself, since it is justifiable to see in him the French equivalent of Goya.   Thus Jean Grenier has established a lineage that passes from Goya, through Daumier, to Rouault.

Daumier, of course, did not witness in his own country such appalling tragedies as the great Aragonese saw in Spain.   He spent only a short time in prison and under conditions which, during the reign of the Citizen-King, could hardly be considered as martyrdom.   He was never exiled.   The creator of the unforgettable «Rue Transnonain» had no experience of vast massacres or the horrors of war.   During the terrible year of 1871 he was consoled, like so many Republicans, by the avenging fate that overtook Badinguet and Ratapoil[5].   He had been haunted by the victims of the July Revolution and various riots, but those of February and even of December 2nd, left him with fewer nightmares than one might suppose.   He was a patriot, it is true, dreaming of revenge even before the «Revanchards[6]» made themselves heard, but above all he was a pacifist.   His vision of the battlefields, of the levies of a licencious soldiery, are magnificent yet somewhat abstract.   Whether he is dealing with doctors, bourgeois or speculators, he is invariably carried away by his inspired imagination. His was a sombre and prophetic genius with none of the naïve optimism of Victor Hugo that left its mark on a whole generation.   In fact, Daumier was a humorist of the gloomy sort who probably suffered from melancholy.   Nowadays, he might tempt the psychoanalysts if he was not known to have been a good fellow in private life, energetic, a hard worker and fundamentally kindly and upright.   Indeed, it must be mentioned that he rarely had occasion to fall into the hands of the Faculty and suffer from the medical incompetence of his day.   Until his final illness that led to such distressing blindness, he had enjoyed good health.   Compared with Stendhal, Flaubert, Baudelaire and even Balzac — who died at the age of fifty — he seems to have had an excellent « physiology ». As this word was considered literary at the time, he himself studied the « physiology» of the Janitress, the Stroller, the Swindler, the Man of Means, Robert Macaire[7] and the Traveller.

The severity with which Daumier treated the medical profession should, therefore, not be ascribed to any personal resentment. His grudge against it was merely part of a grudge against society in general which has struck certain of his biographers and admirers. They have noticed how insensitive was this plebeian, this workingman's son, to the beauty in the lives of the common people, also how chaste and jansenistic in his portrayal of women and his allusions to love. Only one of his pictures — the Allegory he executed for the new Republic — varied on this point, but it was an official commission and is far from being one of his most personal works. His father is said to have been a great lover of poetry. I can detect the artist himself, revealed in his studies of collectors. The reverent gestures of these connoisseurs disclose their emotion, as if he were foreseeing the fanatical enthusiasts of his own lithographic prints.

On the whole, Daumier, like Goya, was a puritan, without being aware of it. But was he entirely unaware? Gavarni immortalized the slender silhouettes of the «Parisiennes» of his day; Constantin Guys conventionalized their elegance; Daumier surveyed this world below with the solemn eyes of the most secular, but also the most suspicious of moralists. A comparison of his lithographs with those of Victor Bassaguet or Célestin Nanteuil shows that he well deserved this austere title.

Being himself an aesthete and a secret libertarian, Baudelaire had great admiration for Guys and he also appreciated the artist of *le Charivari* [8]. However, Daumier himself dreamed of improving mankind by stigmatizing its faults, whereas most of the so-called «realistic» novelists put up very well with these failings, enjoyed the spectacle of them and had no desire for an earthly paradise or a City of the Sun inhabited solely by the just and virtuous. In spite of a few nude compositions that reveal a certain sensuality, or *libido*, Daumier seems to have had little indulgence for the things of the flesh.

This tendency in his character and works explains the rather morose gravity with which he depicts the various classes and professions. Whether he is dealing with the Bourgeoisie, the Law or the medical profession, he pretends to find only monsters among them — a tendency that provoked a doubly unpleasant comment by the Goncourt brothers [9] who wrote of his water-colors : «They're all done with watered India ink, spectrally fantastic, the heads are hideous and often terrifyingly enlarged.» And they went on to recognize wild beasts and Corybants in these peaceable lawyers and worthy doctors! Town doctors, all of them, for he could have known none in the country, and there is no Dr. Benassis in his teratological portrait gallery.

There exists, in fact, for the artist a certain temptation to conceive of the « medical phenomenon » as being somehow anti-natural. To many men, everything connected with illness and inevitably with death, seems apocalyptically hilarious, terrifying or heart-breaking. Perhaps this is one of the ways in which the mind defends itself against painful truths. In the same way, macabre humor has long been one of the mainstays of the theater and of satirical poetry, and there are plenty of examples of nosological humor, since fear can be exorcised by making suffering appear ridiculous. There is a traditional tendency to exaggerate the tyranny imposed on us by our mortal coil. Chamber-pots and clysters have been a subject for jokes ever since these humble objects came into existence. Medicine in both its active and passive aspects — that is, doctors and their patients — was a favorite subject for caricaturists up to the time of Abel Faivre, half a century ago and even more recently for Gus Bofa. Indeed, an erudite study could be written on the comic aspects of medicine in France and the Occident, and even in the Orient, since Arab literature could provide an immense amount of documentation. Because Daumier was a moralist as well as a humorist, his themes were more varied and cruel and he treated them, as Paul Valéry has said, with the severity of a judge, and with profound sadness. The doctors in his engravings are invariably pedantic, vain, avid, egoistic, or hard and indifferent. They personify the inevitable imperfections of a science in constant evolution and which, it must be admitted, was still far from adult in Daumier's day. Great progress had already been made but it was not yet admired and venerated by the wide public that today follows the most esoteric researches with mingled gratitude and reverent terror. Medicine as seen or imagined by Daumier was indeed that of a bygone age. We can measure the distance covered by recalling the abysmal ignorance of the masses a century ago. These good people — whether they represented the talkative men-about-town of the *Tortoni,* Henri Monnier's gossipping housewives or Paul de Kock's little working-girls — were absolutely ignorant of even the most elementary biology. Thus it was an easy matter to caricature the magicians in their black robes and square caps or their frock-coats and white cravattes. Their costume lent them the authority that science still lacked.

What, then, can have been the mental reaction of our ancestors, accustomed as they were to wide-scale mortality, to such irresistible epidemics as pest, cholera or typhus fever? Today, war plays much the same role for us but without having quite the same quality of diabolical fatality. People were haunted by the Angel of Death, in one form or another, and their jokes were an instinctive form of defense. It may be that the gradual triumph of optimism in political philosophy was made possible by scientific discoveries. Daumier's character and artistic calling led him to give expression to this open suspicion and secret apprehension. In his famous picture, *Cholera,* for instance, there are no doctors to be seen. The vision depicted is that of a devastated city in which the corpses will soon be succeeded by their ghosts. It helps us to appreciate the serious side of Molière's *Malade Imaginaire* which deals, not with the traditional matter of comedy, but with the insoluble conflict between man's anxiety and suspect therapeutic expedients. He was not being unjustly spiteful but was expressing the hopes of a heart continually moved to compassion. Comparing Daumier with Molière, Baudelaire praised both of them for the certainty they showed and the way in which they aimed straight at their goal. The idea behind the work of both men is evident and understandable at a glance.

It would not perhaps be going beyond the proper limits of psychological investigation to suggest that Daumier had certain deep-seated tendencies — without going so far as to call them moral predispositions — resulting from his character and the circumstances of his life. Like Michelet and Veuillot[10], he was a son of the people and led a life of arduous labor. The Moloch of journalism undoubtedly devoured part of his mind and body, though without apparently diminishing his genius or deforming his art. His profession did, however, cast on him a certain discredit that for a long time prevented the critics and historians of art, in spite of the protests of such leading spirits as Baudelaire and Balzac, from according him his true place among the great masters. He had numerous and flattering friendships among liberal writers and artists, but until 1871, he had no hope of becoming an official artist. Once this became possible it was too late, and we know that he died in poverty. If it had not been for the tact and generosity of Corot, he could not even have acquired the cottage in Valmondois where he remained, half blind and receiving only a few visitors, until his death. There is a little monument on the banks of the Oise where so many men of letters make their homes today, but this memorial is in the nature of an atonement. We are told that Dr. Vanier, who tended this caricaturist of doctors during his last illness, finding that his pulse was barely perceptible, remarked : « The end has come. » But in reality everything was beginning for Daumier. He was entering a night that was also to be the dawn of a brilliant reputation.

Daumier's genius, as the Goncourts have said, was above all of a fantastic kind, and it is not, perhaps, of much use to search his works for historical and sociological truths. Yet this sort of research is necessary, just as it was in the case of Balzac, who moves us today as a visionary rather than as the observer and chronicler of a bygone world. It was Balzac, in fact, who first proclaimed his faith in Daumier. «There is something of Michelangelo in him», he once declared, and we can judge the truth of his remark by studying a lithographic print entitled *Soup,* about which a whole book could be written and called *Hunger,* or *The Couple,* or *The Human Beast.* There was a certain community of taste and instinct between the two men, who collaborated in their contributions to *la Caricature.* This «Marseillais» and this Gascon (for Balzac's family came from the Aquitaine region) recognized each other's merits. However, the painter lived twenty years longer than the novelist who, in spite of all his trials and financial difficulties, led the life of a wealthy and respected man and successfully courted several ladies of quality. If, as he himself declared, he died of thirty thousand cups of coffee, Daumier may be said to have died of ten thousand drawings and sketches. He inhabited dusty studios or the poorest kind of apartments; he never even attempted to go into business; and he remained faithful to the little dressmaker he married. One can hardly imagine an existence less Balzacian than that of this Balzacian artist. Yet Daumier too created a world parallel to that of everyday life. As Focillon has remarked, «out of the difficult necessities of life, out of fleeting moments, out of innumerable news items and witty retorts, he constructed a Human Comedy, a moral history of the nineteenth century that equals the most immortal monuments of genius». The lithographer was indeed building up, stone by stone, a monument that will never cease to attract visitors and pilgrims. Perhaps the comparison of this little universe with that of reality will throw a light on the genius of its creator. The writings of Balzac were illuminated by the twin torches of religion and the monarchy. Daumier had broken free from these august chains but he by no means shared the optimism of his political friends. He was possessed of an epic and tragic demon which forbade him to share Béranger's[11] attitude. «Even his blasphemies are amusing», remarked Baudelaire, who imagined that it was almost by chance that his drawings sometimes seemed terrifying or distressing. In other words, his jokes were sacrilegious, fundamentally disrespectful and militantly sceptical in regard to all the accepted authorities in this world and the next. Like Hugo, he made frequent use of antithesis, contrasting black and white, good and evil. This was the sort of grandiose Manicheism, combined with the simplicity of the common people, that could inspire both *La Bouche d'Ombre* and *Les Mystères de Paris*. From this point of view, Daumier must be considered as a descendant of the Romantics, in whom he could see only what was banal, trite and — as he might say himself — bourgeois.

It will be easier to understand the motives for his medical prints if we consider his treatment of professions less exposed to diabolical interpretations. His butchers, for instance, suddenly take on the aspect of executioners sacrificing to some perverse divinity. Yet it is hard to excuse him for so constantly denouncing a certain inhuman frigidity in face of suffering but never admitting the heroic abnegation, kindness and charity practised by men far too modest to boast of their good deeds.

The captions to his lithographs are seldom worthy of them. They are generally provided by colorless hacks, though Michelet, who considered him comparable with Tacitus in his power of admonishment and lofty style, once wrote to him : « You shall have all my captions as I turn them out ». Great caricaturists have illustrated incisive phrases provided by others, although Forain [12], who was expert at inventing formulae as brief as they were striking, said he could only do so after his drawing was finished. In this case, the intellectual was subordinated to the visual artist, the moralist swept along in the wake of the painter. In Daumier's day, captions were long, labored and rather too explicative. Those used by Gavarni and Grandville were as unnecessarily lengthy as his own. Perhaps the public was accustomed to greater verbosity at that time. Or perhaps Voltairean conciseness had already degenerated, after having forsaken the drawing-room for the café, the weary aristocrat for the greedy bourgeois. Chamfort's wit, like Rivarol's [13], was as quick as lightning, whereas that of the humorists of sixty years later had become like a will o' the wisp in a fog. Doubtless, it reflected the way people thought and talked and thus constitutes a record of feelings and opinions, as well as of the expressions and even slang then in use, in the same way as the dialogues between Henri Monnier's loose-jacketted, phrygian-capped puppets. The conversations between Daumier's characters are those of the average man, but their attitudes and gestures reveal the eternal essence of mankind : a mankind rather more picturesque and, it is to be hoped, rather worse, than in real life.

It should be noted that Daumier treats his patients nearly as badly as he does his doctors. Since he dealt on several occasions with the theme of the imaginary invalid, we gather that he himself was in good health and had no inferiority complex in regard to his own body. The bourgeois or plebeian patients evoked by his crayon or paintbrush are shown as hopelessly ugly and ridiculous. His women are just as badly treated and one might make various psychological conjectures as to the distaste he seems to feel for the feminine form and the temptations of the flesh. How many poor, stupid, absurd creatures he sacrifices to quack doctors and charlatans of all kinds! How many ignorant women who, like their creator, had a horror of dieting and swallowing any sort of medicine! They represent Daumier's own distrust — a distrust that would be universally shared by the sick today if they were faced with the therapeutic methods of his time.

This bitter observer, this choleric reformer, was equally cruel to nurses, dentists, «must-operate» surgeons, solemn professors, empiricists, oculists, homeopaths, magnetizers, and so on. He railed against and jeered at all their methods : dieting, leeches, cranioscopy, pedantic chemistry and, above all, the absurd arsenal of remedies vaunted by the publicity of the mid-century : dromedary ointment, Arab Racahout, up-to-date clysto-pumps. He may have jeered too at the idea of hygiene and the first attempts at antisepsis by spraying with Labarraque's mixture.

As for the professional failings he stigmatizes with a regret that has been described as full of «tolerant good humor» — there is nothing very startling or unjust in his satire. He exercises it on the vanity, greed, ambition, ignorance and arrogance that can be found in all circles and in any profession. Most of us have had occasion to accuse certain doctors of being as indifferent to suffering as the heads of armies, although the role of the former is to cure and that of the latter to kill, but every intelligent patient realizes that, for a doctor, the truest form of compassion is a correct diagnosis. Yet between two equally sound practitioners, he is bound to prefer a courteous doctor to a surly one, one who is sympathetic to one who is insensitive.

It will be noted that most of Daumier's characters live in cities. The magnificent print entitled *The Sick Peasant* is an exception, and he ignores or spares the country doctor and the Army doctor. His work is undoubtedly inspired by direct observation and by a memory so prodigious that it must be assimilated to the creative power, and which Baudelaire describes as «a marvellous and semi-divine memory that provides him with all his models». We can understand something of the mysterious workings of this splendid faculty by recalling that Daumier admitted he had never made a sketch from life. He drew from memory and had an extraordinary gift for stylizing on the spot whatever his eyes recorded. This gift perhaps explains the elegance and precision of his line, the force of his chiaroscuro, the originality and variety of his compositions and the surety with which he poses his figures. All these qualities put him in a class apart from the best-known of his contemporaries, Raffet and Traviès, and their successors, Steinlen, Anquetin and Forain. He is surpassed only by Toulouse-Lautrec, who was not merely a humorist.

Furthermore, like Rembrandt who had so great an influence on him, Daumier had such a strong feeling for volume that he must be counted among the masters of sculptural drawing. His skillful modelling, like that of Degas, confirms the impression that he could have been a great sculptor. In these examples of two-dimensional art we see the same tendency to repeat and transform a pitilessly-observed reality. In his medical scenes, as in all his satires, he has created an unforgettable world in which light and shade compose a true «Sur-reality». As Focillon so well remarks : «In his finest pages he amplifies forms till they appear colossal, while at the same time he seems to simplify the modelling so as to reveal the full eloquence of his forms. Thus this illustrator of leaflets lived in a constant atmosphere of grandeur.»

When Daumier depicts sick men, haunted and assailed by sprites and goblins, he might be a direct descendant of Breughel and Jérôme Bosch. When he transforms his political opponents, Dr. Prunelle and Dr. Véron, into monstrous allegories, he literally ceases to see them in their terrestrial aspect and recreates them in the form of mythic figures. Even in his political polemics he knew how to sublimate the most banal metaphors and banish all vulgarity from his comments. Indeed, if he had not been a journalist by profession, he might have produced only masterpieces. And even as it was, working as he did at top speed and for an audience of dubious taste, he did indeed produce a number of pathetic or terrifying masterpieces, for example, in his series on *Painful Moments in Life,* on the page which shows simply a dentist with his patient. Here, the construction and powerful simplicity of the drawing raise the subject to the level of the classic themes of torture, fear and human passivity. In the same way, the famous composition, *Doctors and Death,* with its movement of sombre draperies, is only a drawing, yet it reveals an almost abstract conflict between Pride and Ferocity such as the morality plays of the sixteenth century used to portray. The doctors in robes and neckbands, the books of wizardry, the peremptory gestures, the faces that are almost as graphic as they are plastic, all seem to proceed from the mind of a poet rather than the memory of an artist. Perhaps this sort of magic was a legacy from his father who, though he was a laborer as

18

humble as that of Watteau, had been intoxicated by poetry. When the artist imagined a man throwing his dog into the water, he was not illustrating a banal event but staging an example of pure murder, unpunished, semi-legal, yet which would bring inexpiable shame and remorse on its perpetrator. Scholars contest the authenticity of this work, but surely no other than Daumier could have imagined such a fable, the moral of which is so closely related to his indictment of unconscientious doctors : « Thou shalt not trifle with death. »

*
* *

Did he use real doctors as his models before conjuring them away to leave place for their fictitious and unflattering archetypes? Or did he perhaps get all this spiteful information from Dr. Fabre for whom he illustrated a work entitled *Medical Nemesis* that was richer in alexandrine lines than in poetry and which Baudelaire called «a rather bad work»?

It was in his role as an Orleanist deputy that Daumier portrayed Dr. Prunelle, the mayor of Lyons, as pot-bellied and shaggy-haired. He was fond of Eugène Sue[14], who had been a surgeon in the navy and whose works he could have illustrated so magnificently. But he did not spare the famous surgeon J.-B. Dumas, professor at the University of Medicine, who had been elected senator and rendered great service to Paris as a town councillor. He was an official personage and thus automatically an enemy for this intransigent rebel. As for Dr. Véron, we know how he was treated in this carnaval of victims. He was even attacked by the virtuous Provençal for his feminine conquests, for his liaisons with Rachel and Marie Duplessis[15]. Daumier's portraits showed him as a sort of monster, dressed or undressed in a hundred different ways, but he did not practice as a doctor and was only given the title out of politeness. Although there were innumerable stories of his vulgarity, cupidity and insolence, it was certainly because he was editor of *le Constitutionnel* and Director of the *Opéra* that Daumier portrayed him as one of the selfish, pleasure-seeking bourgeois he held in horror.

According to those who knew him, the engraver of *le Charivari* did not know much about medicine. He jeered at Gall's ideas on phrenology, yet, like Lavater's theories on physiology, they may well have helped him to make his heads and faces so expressive. Perhaps he knew some of the German doctors who had been prospering in Paris since the Restoration, and notably the strange and suspect Dr. Koreff, who was part miracle-worker, part spy, as well as hypnotiser, and who treated the *Dame aux Camélias,* Liszt, A. de Custine and others

19

with his peculiar methods. Quacks always have luck in Paris, wherever they come from and whatever their specialty. Snobbishness, curiosity and idle talk are sure to bring them patients. Perhaps Koreff, a character who might have stepped out of the Tales of Hoffmann, was partly responsible for the picture Daumier invented, with or without Fabre's help, of the medical world. Some twenty lithographic prints remind us of him rather than of innumerable honest and prudent practitioners. It was of him that Grandville, Daumier's colleague and contemporary, was thinking when he too tried his hand at macabre fantasy.

*
* *

Perhaps we shall find it easier to judge Daumier's work if we compare it for a moment with that of the writers of his day, glance at some of their opinions on it and consider to what extent he resembled them. One cannot, indeed, imagine him painting the austere portraits of Dr. Benassis or Dr. Bianchon. Neither the infinitely moving story of *La Messe de l'Athée* nor the humanitarian apostolate of *Le Médecin de campagne* could have been included in his album. Balzac, unlike Daumier, had known doctors worthy of his full respect.

Curiously enough, it is rather in the Goncourts' *Journal* that images resembling those of Daumier are to be found : the transfer to the hospital of «La Pitié» of a dying old woman; the apocalyptic hospital scenes that reappeared later in *Sœur Philomène,* the theme of which was provided by their friend Louis Bouillat, an ex-medical student; the picturesque souvenirs of Ricord; certain dissertations on the inhumanity into which they believed medicine would gradually sink as it became more and more scientific and industrialized. The Goncourts, or rather the elder of them, who survived his brother, understood Daumier so well that we may wonder if he did not exercise an influence over these great visual artists.

If we consider the medical world with which painters and writers were familiar between the fall of the Empire and the Third Republic, we shall see that it was not the pandemonium invented by Daumier's satiric wit and creative genius, and which must not be confused with the average qualities of an observer or chronicler. Stendhal, for instance, had good reason, since his youthful love-affairs, for consulting numerous doctors. He came of a medical family, through the Gagnons, and perhaps inherited from them his epicurism, his rationalism and a facile respect for the sons of Hippocrates, as they were called at the beginning of the century. His private diary shows him in Rouen, Milan, Pavia, Paris, visiting doctors and healers, suffering from an endless series of giddiness, fever and neuralgia. We can deduce from them that H. Beyle[16] was a chronic semi-invalid and docile patient. He expresses special consideration for Dr. Edwards, the renowned ethnologist, for Dr. Koreff, whom he would have done better to distrust, and for Dr. Prévost of Geneva who he believed had alleviated his arthritis. One could draw up a whole list of the doctors he held in honor, not forgetting Henri Martineau, who treated his memory so lovingly, after his death.

A study of this list would show how differently the neurotic Beyle and the healthy Daumier viewed this subject. Perhaps writers are more delicate than painters and tend to be more grateful and timid in regard to their doctors. Among the endless parallels that could be drawn up on this subject, Sainte-Beuve must not be forgotten for, like his own Joseph Delorme, he was an ex-medical student[17]. He had studied with Dupuytren and Richerand and retained a sincere affection for the physiologists and ideologists he had known in his youth. It was as a patient, however, that he met Ricord. Whereas Stendhal made certain reservations, he never had praise enough for the intelligence, culture and self-abnegation of doctors. If he ever saw Daumier's caricatures, he certainly would not have needed to ask himself if the models really resembled their portraits. As a literary historian he knew well that medicine was far from being an exact science at that time and was thus constantly exposed to satire, especially when the prosperity of its practitioners contrasted sharply with the misery of men of letters.

Mérimée[18], who was a realist, suffered continually from chronic illness and complained of spasms, migraines, breathlessness and rhumatism. In medical matters, his god seems to have been the illustrious Bretonneau and his demi-god Professor Hippolyte Royer-Collard, and he arranged for the latter to be treated by the former. He himself consulted therapeutists in Cannes, Montpellier and Paris for his incurable asthma. Like Stendhal, the best treatment he received from the hands of any doctor was that given after his death and, in his case, he owes it to the scholarly Dr. Maurice Parturier.

What did Flaubert[19], who was a surgeon's son and had a poor constitution, think about doctors? He occasionally railed against the incompetence of medicine in general and certain practitioners in particular, but, like his friend Bouilhet, he considered medicine the most dramatic of all professions and believed it demanded the feeling for truth which he often found lacking in poets. There is nothing comic about his Charles Bovary, that unhappy husband and unlucky health officer, and Flaubert certainly understood more than Daumier of the anguish that besets every doctor worthy of the name and the secret generosity they practice every day.   On the subject of Flaubert, I should regret not to recall some of the admirable features from which he builds up the portrait of Dr. Larivière, whose qualities were less rare than the satirists imagined : «He belonged to that generation of philosophic practitioners who have a fanatical devotion to their art and exercised it with enthusiasm and sagacity...   He disdained, I imagine, official titles and academic honors; he was hospitable, liberal-minded, paternal towards the poor and good without believing in the existence of goodness.   He might have passed for a saint if he had not been feared like the devil for his biting wit...   His eyes were even more piercing than his lancets.   They looked straight into the soul and disarticulated the lies concealed beneath reticence and excuses...»

Few of us, perhaps, unite in ourselves so many admirable qualities.   However, I should like to dedicate these lines, with all the perspicacity that underlies their generosity and the profound truths they express with such elegance, to the best among those I have encountered, and their number is far from being insignificant.   May they recognize themselves in this radiant image!

If we consider the fundamental resemblance or dissemblance between Daumier's opinions and those of the writers I have chosen for mention because they bear witness to their century or to two generations within it, and because they had dealings with doctors, we shall see that, although some of them had great critical intelligence and showed a good deal of scepticism and deference to public opinion, they are reassuring after Daumier's gloomy portrayals.   None of them has depicted the medical profession as the sorry carnival or grotesque dance of death that Daumier created for the delectation of his admirers, among whom must be counted numerous doctors.

Daumier has been compared to Rabelais, Molière and Balzac.   His was an epic form of genius and more lyrical than it appears to the casual eye.   Besides the masterpieces that are a sufficient justification in themselves, he has left us an immense documentation on the ideal of the common man in regard to Medicine.   It is a nostalgic ideal, a dream — sometimes a nightmare — through which there winds a procession of hideous, deformed and sublimated doctors and patients who reveal, perhaps unconsciously, less bitterness than an irremediable regret that men can be tended in sickness only by other men.

As for the latter, our beloved Montaigne[20], who refused to admit that his respect for doctors arose only from need of their services, added : «I hold doctors in esteem, not in order to set a good example, nor out of necessity, but for love of themselves, since I have seen among them many honest men, worthy to be loved.» The pleasure so many doctors take in Daumier's harsh works comes perhaps from the fact that all have met examples of ignorant, unqualified and boastful colleagues who thoroughly justify them.

Daumier was accorded his rightful place by Balzac, Delacroix, Corot, Baudelaire and Michelet during his lifetime, and posterity soon followed suit. It is a pleasure to read the brilliant and expert tributes of our own contemporaries. «Here is Daumier's universe», writes Henri Focillon, «or rather, certain aspects of it which reveal some of the superlative faculties of the man himself — the immense scope of his work, the force with which he endows the particular and temporary with general and lasting significance; the popular and universal accent of his humor, which, like that of Molière, anyone can understand, and finally, his noble bitterness and generous heart. In other words, he is of truly male lineage, unlike so many delightful artists, endowed with the most seductive charms with which they clothe even their cynicism, so that it appears charming in its turn.» Claude Roger-Marx considers that Daumier was one of the men who, in the words of Delacroix, are born into the world ready and fully-armed, and says of him : «Lies, Envy, Egoism, Old Age, are boldly mocked from his chiaroscuro, but the force of these compositions is such that we could easily ignore the themes that serve as their pretext and reserve all our admiration for the moving form, the epic line detached with such surety from the confused tumult of reality, the splendid conflict of light and shade, and, at the very heart of this apparent mobility, the supreme balance which reveals itself, from the plastic point of view, as the other aspect of Daumier's vast wisdom.»

Finally, there is Paul Valéry, who began by saying rather unenthusiastically that «a work of art that does not reduce us to silence can be of little value». But he agreed to write about Daumier all the same, and concluded a fine study by remarking that «he is the great historian of this period : it is not in the books that set out to deal with it that you will find the grocers, the simpletons, the swindlers, the men of law, the employees and the whole living matter of this mediocre age that was content with its mediocrity.

«In the end, he fell in love with Don Quixote...»

HENRI MONDOR

NOTES

1) The celebrated play, *Knock*, by Jules Romains, has been one of the most successful productions of the contemporary French theater. Its main character is a doctor who might be the great-grandson of one of Daumier's pompous charlatans.

2) Paul-Louis Courier (1772-1825), was noted for the biting wit of his political polemics.

3) Henri Monnier (1805-1877), writer and caricaturist, whose *Scènes populaires* form a caustic comment-ary on his times. He created the character of Joseph Prudhomme, the archetype of the early 19th century bourgeois.

4) Joseph Méry (1798-1865), caused considerable annoyance and even moral damage to the Restau-ration Government by his satiric poems.

5) « Badinguet » was the nickname given to Napoleon III and probably taken from the caption to one of Gavarni's lithographs. — « Ratapoil » was a nickname used to describe a partisan of extreme mili-tarism and nationalism — in fact, rather what we should today call a Fascist.

6) « Revanchards » : term used to describe the people who, after the defeat of 1870, urged for a new war against Prussia to restore the honor of France.

7) Robert Macaire was a type of audacious rascal invented by the authors of a melodrama called *L'Auberge des Adrets* and popularized by the famous actor, Frédérick Lemaître. Daumier's caricatures show him successively in the guise of a banker, barrister, journalist, etc.

8) *Le Charivari* was a satirical review founded in 1832, to which many of the wittiest writers and illustrators of the day were contributors.

9) The brothers Edmond and Jules Huot de Goncourt collaborated till the death of Jules in 1870 in novels in the « naturalist » style and in studies in aesthetics. Nowadays, they are chiefly known for the private diary in which they noted the sayings and doings of the outstanding literary and artistic figures of the day, and for the « Académie Goncourt », founded by Edmond de Goncourt and which attributes a yearly prize for the best French novel.

10) Jules Michelet (1798-1874), a celebrated historian of liberal and humanitarian tendencies. — Louis-François Veuillot (1813-1883), violent « ultra » catholic polemist who founded the journal *l'Univers* and left a voluminous and brilliant correspondence.

11) Pierre-Jean de Béranger (1780-1857), composer of popular songs, who aspired to be the champion of the People.

12) Jean-Louis Forain (1852-1931), chiefly known for his satiric drawings, aimed largely at the Law.

13) Nicolas-Sébastien Roch, commonly called de Chamfort (1741-1794). His epigrams made him greatly feared in his own day and his « maxims » are still widely quoted. — Antoine Rivaroli, commonly known as the Comte de Rivarol (1753-1801), one of the last representatives of Monarchic society at the end of the 18th century, is still a byeword for epigrams so witty that his fame has come down to posterity in spite of the fact that he left no written work of any note.

14) Eugène Sue (1804-1857), author of the famous *Mystères de Paris* that kept the French reading public breathless with excitement in 1842.

15) Rachel (1820-1858), whose real name was Elisa Félix, was perhaps the most famous tragic actress of her day. — Marie Duplessis (in reality Alphonsine Plessis) [1824-1847], had a short but ardent career and was immortalized by the younger Alexandre Dumas, as *La Dame aux Camélias*.

16) Henri Beyle (1783-1842), was the real name of the novelist Stendhal, the celebrated author of *Le Rouge et le Noir, La Chartreuse de Parme*, etc.

17) Charles-Augustin Sainte-Beuve (1804-1869), chiefly remembered as a literary critic, used the pseudonym « Joseph Delorme » at the beginning of his career.

18) Prosper Mérimée (1803-1870), was the author of numerous novels and short stories, notably *Carmen*, from which Bizet composed his opera.

19) Gustave Flaubert (1821-1880), one of the finest French novelists of the 19th century, author of *Madame Bovary, Salammbô, Bouvard et Pécuchet, L'Éducation Sentimentale*, etc. Charles Bovary is one of the principal characters in the first-mentioned novel.

20) Michel-Eyquem de Montaigne (1533-1592), author of the famous *Essays*, philosopher and moralist.

No. 1. *Mr. Prune*

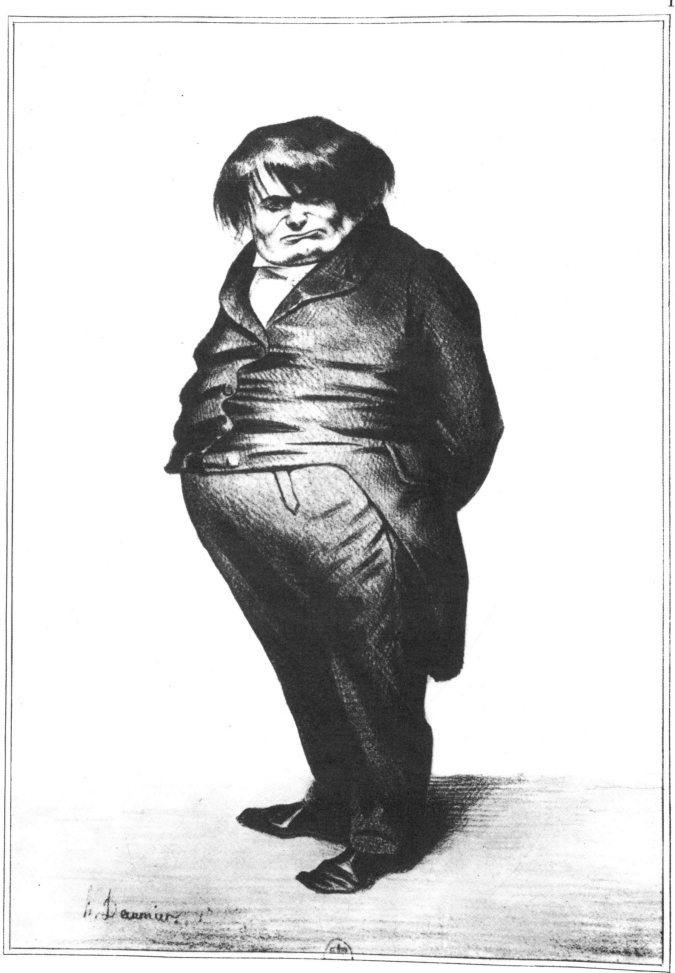

Mr PRUNE.

No. 2.   *Midwife*

Mme de la Piçonnerie, sworn midwife, takes in paying guests for a just price.

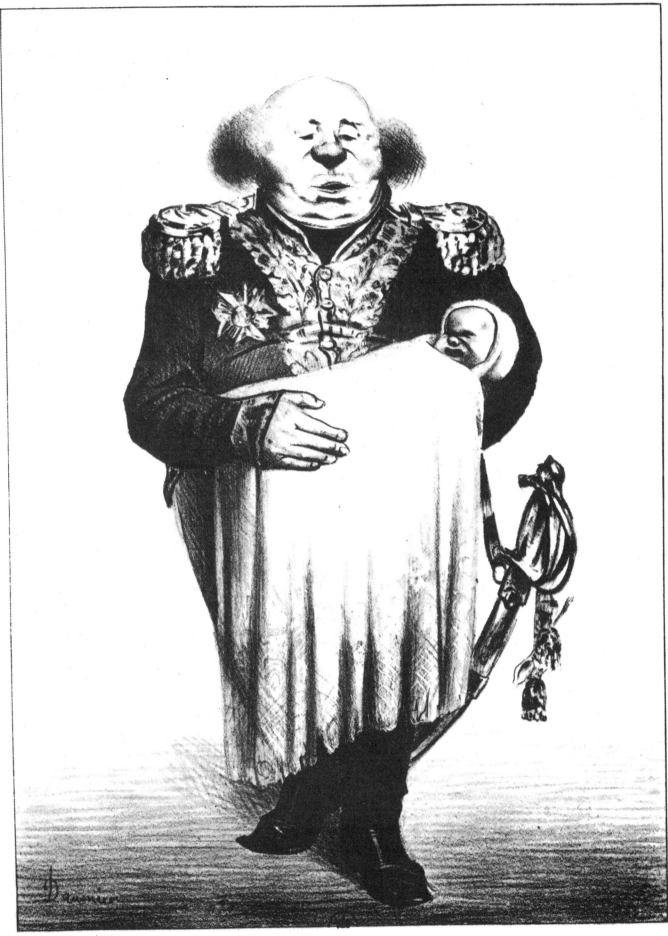

chez Aubert galerie vero dodat.

Mme de la Piçonnerie, accoucheuse jurée, prend des pensionnaires à juste prix.

No. 3.   *The Sick Man*

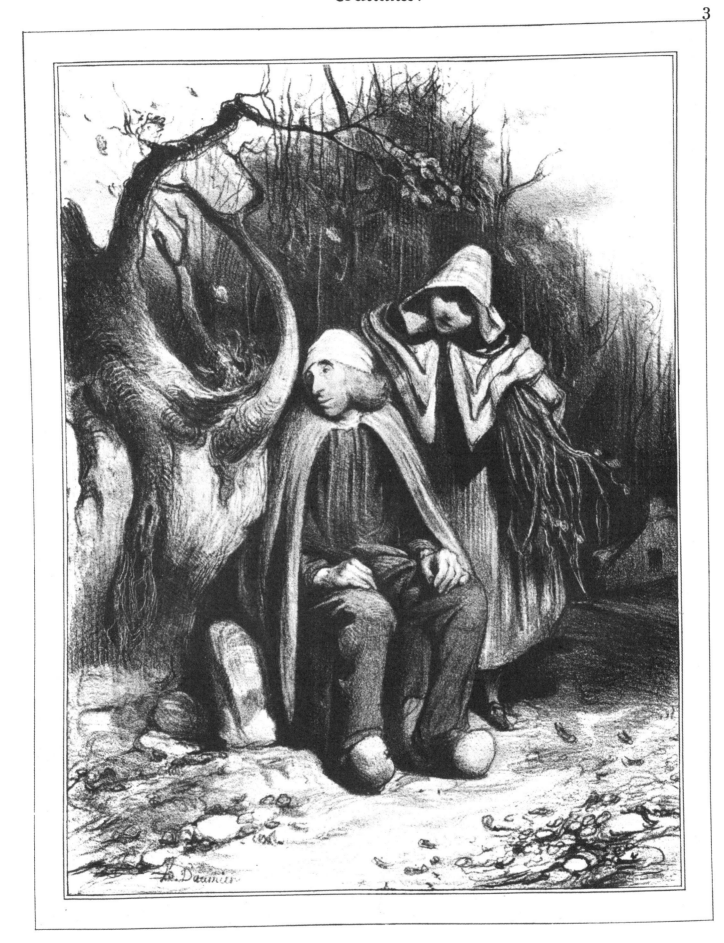

LE MALADE

No. 4. *Medicine*

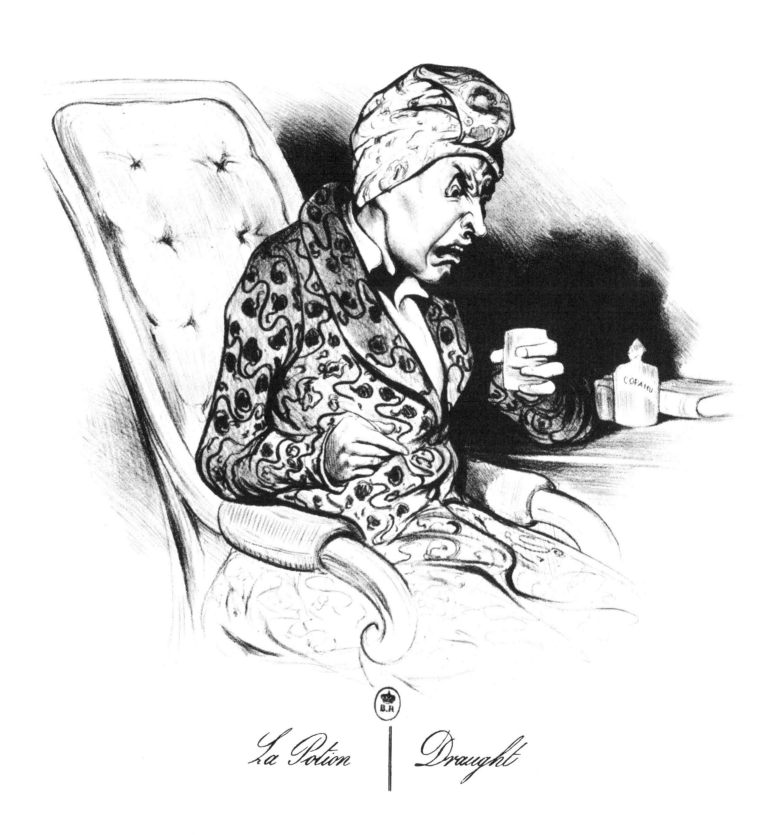

La Potion | Draught

No. 5.

« Today, put in the column of Paris News : The noted doctor Blaguefort (play on words : blague *meaning a trick*) has just succumbed to an attack of the disease that is now fashionable. This news has plunged the capital into deep sadness. Tomorrow, you will insert a correction : We have learned with pleasure that the noted Doctor Blaguefort has completely recovered and resumed his consultations. Every week put in a different little notice and come around each month for payment. »

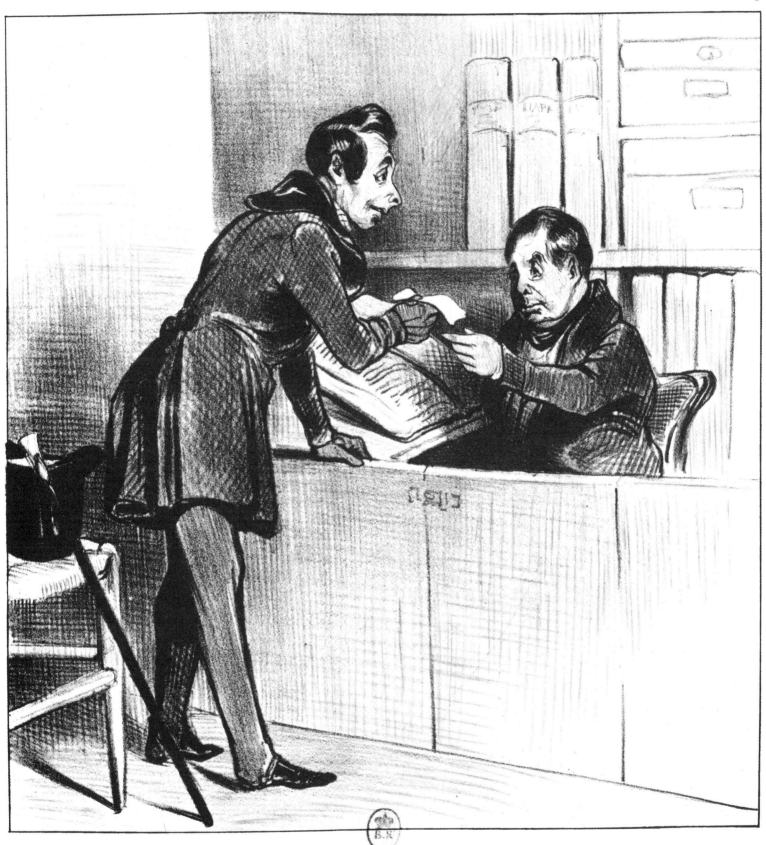

Vous mettrez aujourd'hui, dans les faits Paris : Le célèbre Docteur Blaguefort vient de succomber
à une atteinte de la maladie à la mode. Cette nouvelle a plongé la capitale dans une profonde douleur.
Demain, vous mettrez entre filets : Nous apprenons avec plaisir que le célèbre Docteur Blaguefort
est parfaitement rétabli et reprend le cours de ses consultations. Mettez toutes les semaines une
petite réclame de forme variée et faites recevoir chez moi tous les mois.

No. 6.   *Robert Macaire Philanthropist*

« *You see, Bertrand, we are moralists in actions (play on words : actions also means stocks and bonds)… in actions that cost, naturally, 2 5 0 francs ! We will treat the stockholders free of charge ; you will purge them, I will bleed them.* »

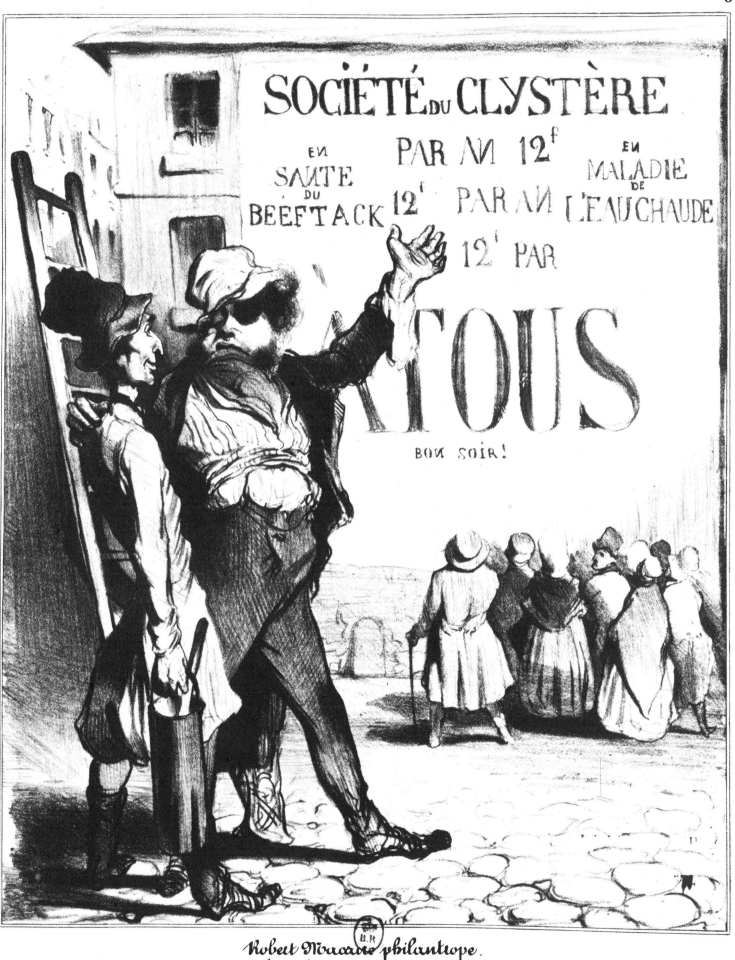

6

Robert Macaire philantrope.

Vois tu, Bertrand, nous faisons là de la morale en actions...... en actions de 250 francs bien
entendu!.— Nous soignerons les actionnaires gratis, tu les purgeras, moi, je les saignerai.

No. 7.   *The Doctor Robert Macaire*

« For heaven's sake, don't take this sickness lightly!... Believe me, drink water, lots of water... rub the bones of your legs... and come to see me often... that won't impoverish you... my consultations are free... Now, you owe me 20 francs for these two bottles... (this includes 10 centimes deposit on each container). »

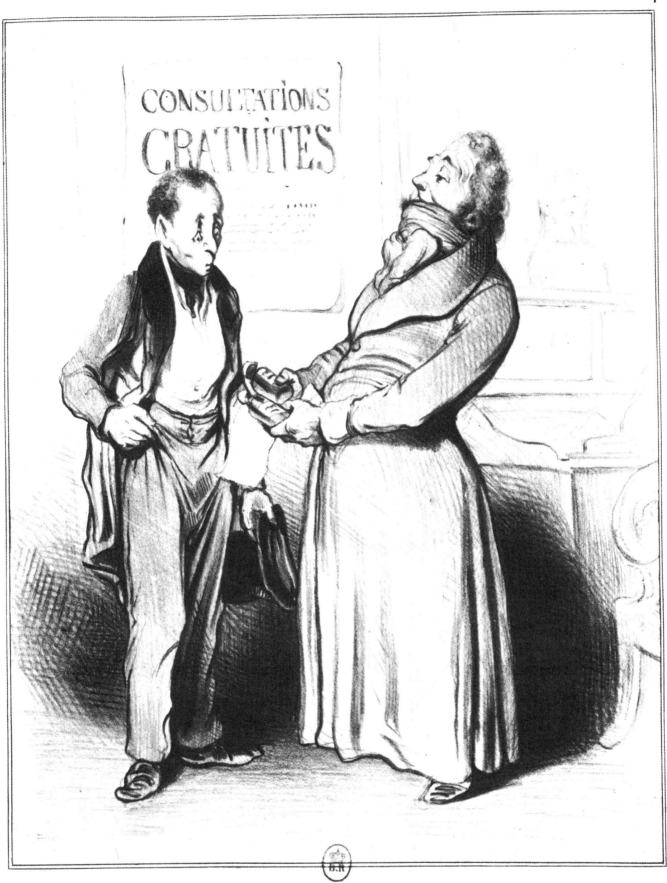

7

Diable! ne plaisantez pas avec cette maladie!...... Croyez moi, buvez de l'eau, beaucoup d'eau! Frottez vous les os des jambes et revenez me voir souvent, ça ne vous ruinera pas mes consultations sont gratuites... ...... Vous me devez 20ˢ pour ces deux bouteilles (On reprend le verre pour 10 centimes)

No. 8.   *Apothecary and Druggist*

«My dear Boniface, it took an apothecary in the old days forty years to assure himself an annual income of 2.000 francs. You walked, we fly (volons : an untranslatable play on words, meaning both fly *and* steal*). — But how do you manage ? — We take some suet, crushed brick or starch, we call it Onicophane Ointment, or Racabout, or Nafé, or Osmaniglou, or any gibberish, then we advertise, send out prospectuses and circulars... and in 10 years we've made a million... We make a frontal attack on Fortune. You used to approach from the wrong side ! »*

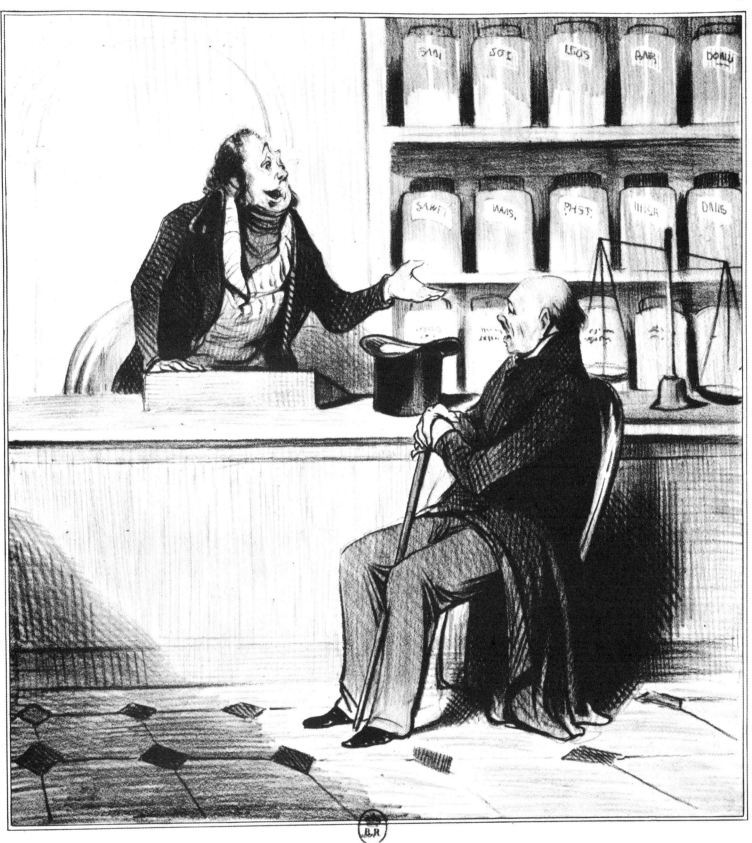

8

Apothicaire ou Pharmacien.

Mon cher Boniface, il fallait autrefois à un apothicaire quarante ans pour gagner 2000 f. de rentes.....
.....vous marchiez nous volons nous! — Mais comment faites vous donc? — Nous prenons du suif, de la
brique pilée ou de l'amidon, nous appelons ça pâte Onicophane, Racahout, Nafé, Osmaniglou ou de tout autre nom
plus ou moins charabia, nous faisons des annonces, des prospectus, des circulaires et en dix ans nous réalisons un
million..... Il faut attaquer la fortune en face, vous la prenez du mauvais côté!!

No. 9.   *A Licensed Oculist*

«*Listen, Mr. Macaire, for six months now you've been promising me wonders with your marvelous eye-wash, and still I'm blind. It ends up by costing me dear, my money is melting away, and that's all I see... — Well, at least that's something; keep on, and you'll get to where you'll see cleardy... (aside) in your pocket book.*»

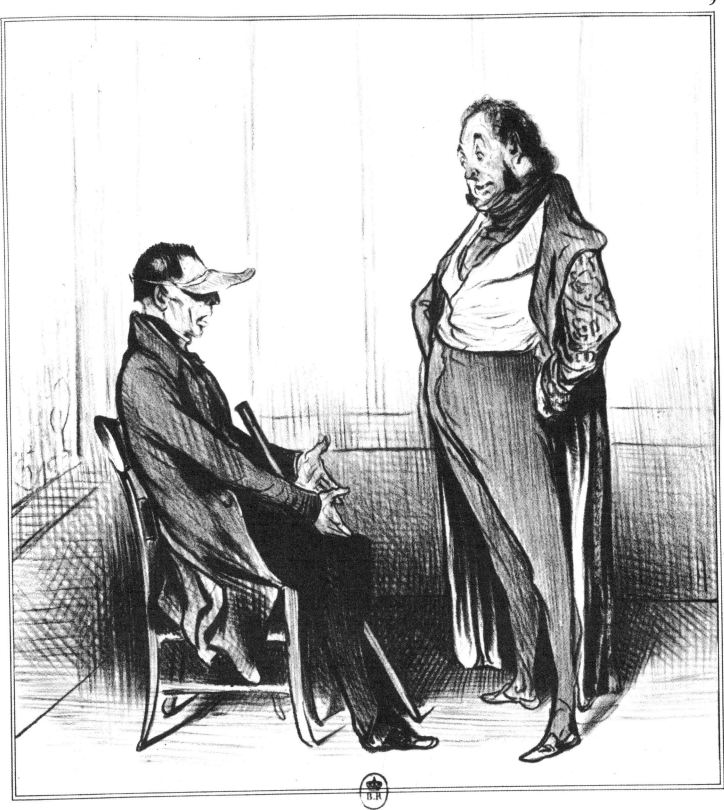

9

Un Oculiste breveté.

Ah! ça, Monsieur Macaire, depuis six mois vous me lassinez avec votre eau merveilleuse et je suis toujours aveugle. Cela finit par me couter bien cher, mon argent s'en va, c'est tout ce que je vois......Hé bien! c'est déja quelque chose; continuez, vous finirez par y voir clair. .....(à Part) dans votre bourse.

No. 10. *Robert Macaire, the Dentist*

«Great God, Doctor, you've pulled out two good teeth and left two bad ones... (Dentist aside) — I'll be damned!... (Aloud). Of course I did, for good reasons. There'll be plenty of time to pull out the bad ones... As for the others, they would eventually have spoiled and caused you pain... A dental plate never hurts, and it's right in style. Everybody's wearing one.»

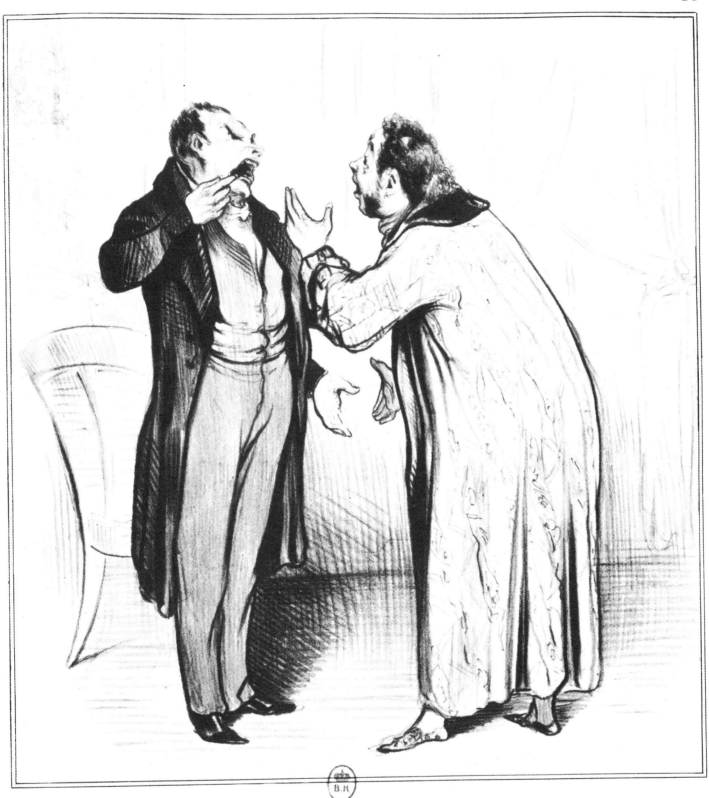

10

Robert Macaire Dentiste.

Sac bleu! Mr le dentiste, vous m'avez arraché deux bonnes dents et vous avez laissé les deux mauvaises . . . . . (Rob. M. à part) Diable!!.. (haut) sans doute! et j'avais mes raisons. . . . . nous sommes toujours à temps d'arracher les mauvaises. . . quand aux autres, elles auraient fini par se gâter et par vous faire mal. . . Un ratelier postiche ne vous fera jamais souffrir, et c'est bien meilleur genre, on ne porte plus que ça.

No. 11.   *Dr. Robert Macaire's clinic*

«*There you are, gentlemen, you've seen this operation, that everyone said was impossible, performed with complete success... — But, Doctor, the patient's dead... — What of it! She would have died anyway even without the operation.*»

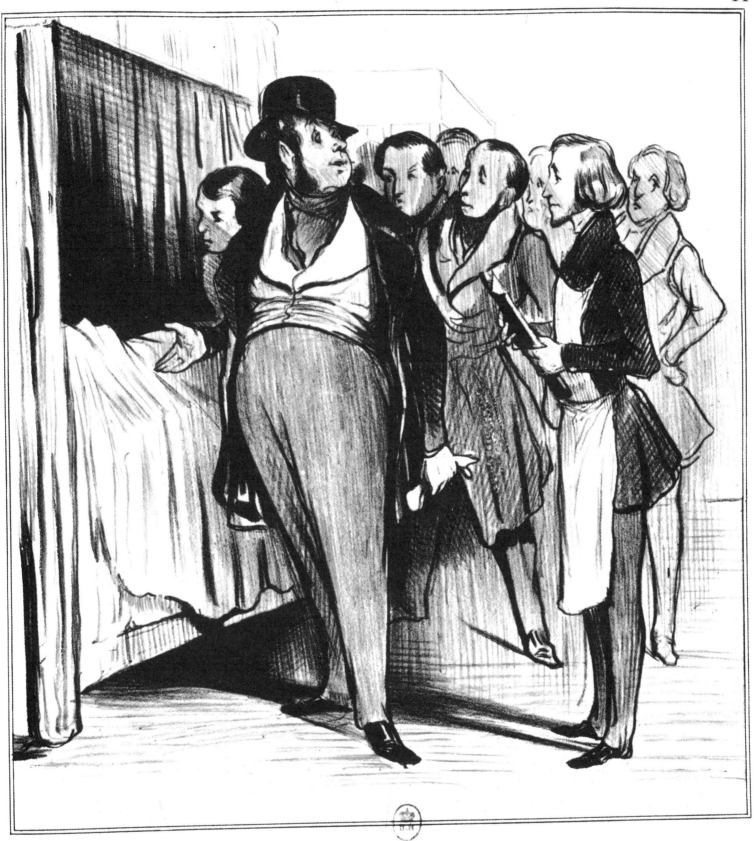

11

Clinique du Docteur Robert - Macaire.

Hé bien ! Messieurs, vous l'avez vû, cette opération qu'on disait impossible a parfaitement réussi !... — Mais, monsieur, la malade est morte...... — Qu'importe ! Elle serait bien plus morte sans l'opération.

No. 12.   *Take this release to the papers*

A gentleman from the provinces after having by mistake swallowed a pouch (play on words : Avaler une blague means also to be taken in), and become suddenly bald and insolvent, the famous Doctor Robert Macaire concluded that pouches (tricks) which ruin some, should, according to 'omiopathy' (for homeopathy), enrich others. The treatment has proved completely successful for him. A hint to the wigs.

« And, as I am named in this article, tomorrow, in accordance with the law of the ninth of September 1835, I shall demand insertion of the following letter.

To the Editor,...   I must request that you publish in your paper the fact that I am not the source of the article, mentioning my name, that you published yesterday. I do cure baldness (one, rue Belle Charge [Belle Charge means high fee]), but I treat it by a different method than that you indicated. Yours truly, Robert Macaire. 1, rue Belle Charge. »

12

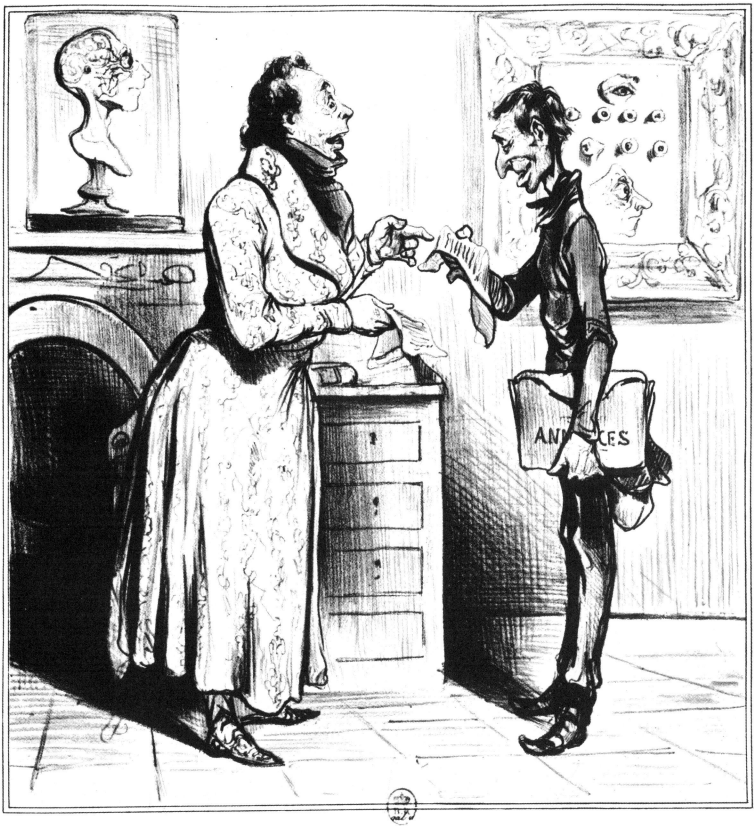

Tu vas porter cette note aux journaux.

Un provincial ayant par mégarde avalé une blague, devint subitement chauve et impoyable, le célèbre Docteur **Robert-Macaire** en conclut que les blagues ruinant les uns doivent, d'après le système omœpathique, enrichir les autres. Le traitement lui a complètement réussi. Avis aux pontugas.

Et comme je suis nommé, dans cet article, demain, en vertu de la loi du 9 7bre 1835, je réclamerai l'insertion de la lettre que voici.

Monsieur le Rédacteur,
Je vous prie de déclarer que vous ne tenez pas de moi l'article dans lequel vous m'avez nommé hier, je m'occupe il est vrai de guérir la calvitie (rue Belle chasse N:1) mais je la traite pas un autre moyen que celui dont vous parlez.
J'ai l'honneur etc.
Robert-Macaire (rue Belle-chasse, N:1)

No. 13.

«*Listen carefully! If you're asked for* muslim Rachout, *to fatten up all kinds of sultanas, for* Arabian nafé *for suckling children of all ages, for* Oriental Kaiffa *to cure gastritis and corns, for* Teribronne *to stop vomiting, for* Amandine, Hindustani, Osman Igloo, Paraguay-Roux, Salep Chocolate, Hypocrasse, White Mustard *for black moods, tooth-ache and deviations in height,* or Giant Cabbage-seed, *you'll find it in this bag, the same one for them all, make no mistake!!! and give it to 'em in the form of a powder, a paste, a solution or pellets, as you see fit. — Gee, what kind o' pellets are they, anyway? They're fool pellets of the best quality. — Wonderful! Wonderful!*»

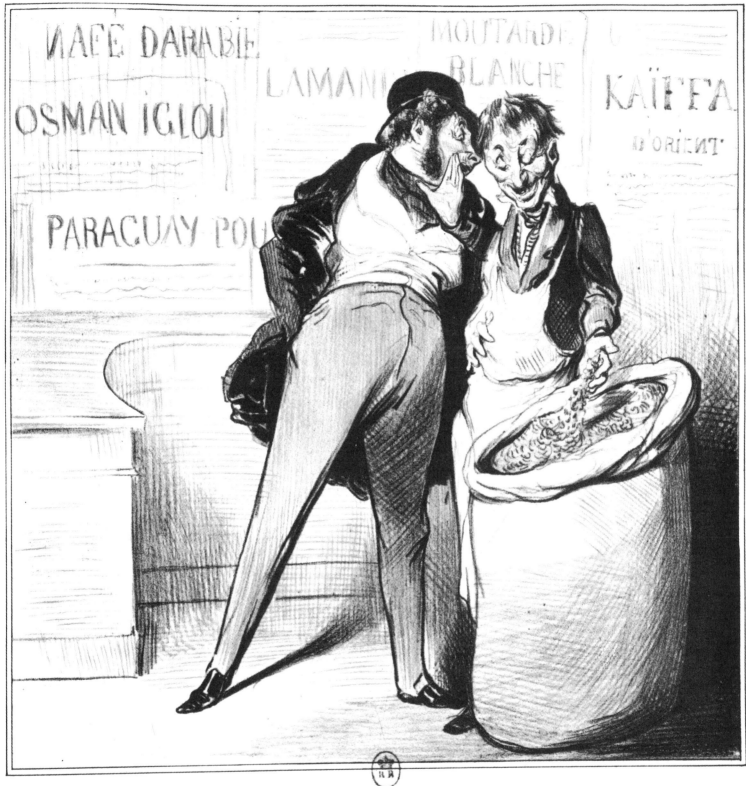

13

Fais bien attention !! Si l'on te demande du Rachaour des arabes pour l'engraissement de toute espèce de sultanes, du Nafé d'arabie pour l'allaitement des enfans de tout âge, du Kaïffa d'orient pour les gastrites et les cors aux pieds, du Teriobronne pour les vomissemens, de l'Amandine, de l'Indostane, de l'Osman-Iglou, du Paraguay-Roux, de la Criosote, du Chocolat au Salep, de l'hypocras, de la Moutarde blanche pour les humeurs noires, les maux de dents et les déviations de la taille, de la Graine de choux colossal tu prendras dans ce sac, toujours dans le même, ne vas pas te tromper !!!! et tu serviras cela en poudre, en pâte, en liqueur ou en graine, suivant ton idée. — Diable, que que c'est donc, que c'te graine là ?... — C'est de la graine de niais première qualité. — Fameux ! fameux !!!!

No. 14.

« The public, old fellow, is stupid... We bleed it, we physic it to death, and it's not satisfied... It wants a change... All right, let's give it something new, by becoming homœopaths... Similia similibus. » — Bertrand : Amen ! — Look, here's a prescription that sums up the system : Take a tiny grain of... nothing at all... separate it into 10 million molecules... throw one, just one of these ten-millionth parts into the river... stir, until well mixed... let it sleep several hours... fill a pail with this healing water... filter... dilute with twenty parts of ordinary water... and wet the tongue with it every morning before breakfast. — Is that all? — Yes... damn it, I forgot the most important part : Pay for this prescription. »

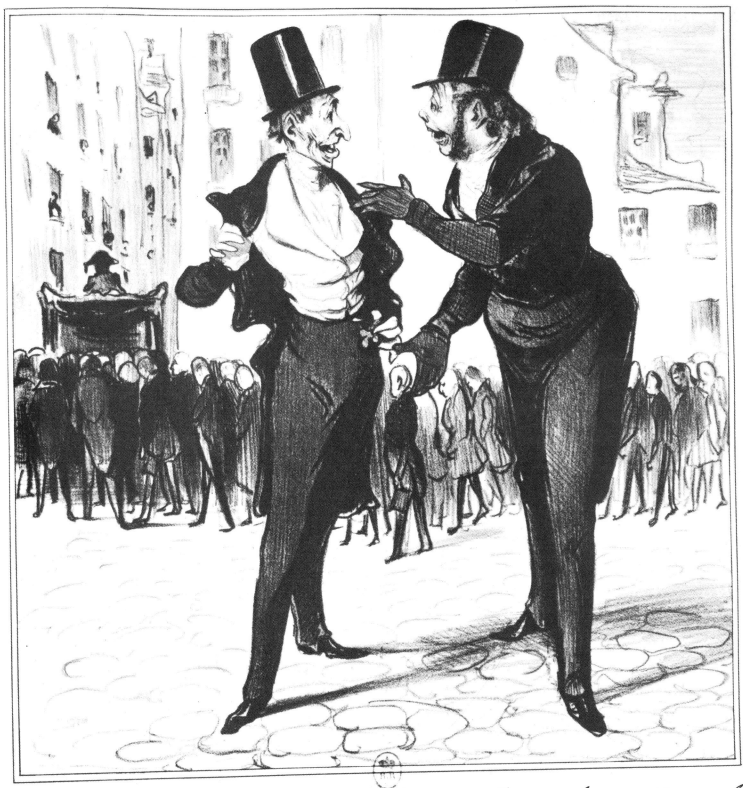

14

Le public, mon cher, le public est stupide.... nous le saignons à blanc, nous le purgeons à mort, il n'est pas content.... il veut du nouveau.... donnons lui en, morbleu, du nouveau! faisons nous homœopates.... Similia similibus. —(Bertrand) Amen! — Tiens, voici une ordonnance qui résume le système. Prendre un pour petit grain de .... de rien du tout .... le couper en dix millions de mollécules .... jeter une .... une seule! de ces dix millionnièmes parties dans la rivière .... remuer, remuer, triturer beaucoup .... laisser infuser quelques heures .... puiser un sceau de cette eau bienfaisante.... la filtrer .... la couper avec 20 parties d'eau ordinaire et s'en humecter la langue tous les matins, à jeun .... Voila! — Est-ce tout? — Oui.... Ah! diable! j'oubliai le principal .... Payer la présente ordonnance.

No. 15.   *How to cure the cramps*

«Mr. Macaire, my good friend, don't make me miss this performance, I need it badly. — Ah, my friend, I can't play, I'm in such pain... — Try, I beg you... the public is demanding you; they're shouting, threatening, ready to rip out the seats. I'll have to return their money... Come, I'll double your bonus. — Oh, Oh, heat some towels... bring some hot wine, heat the towels. — I'll triple your bonus. — Keep the heat on... keep heating the towels. — We'll share the box office receipts. — We'll share the box office receipts? Up with the curtain. The farce is ended, the drama begins...»

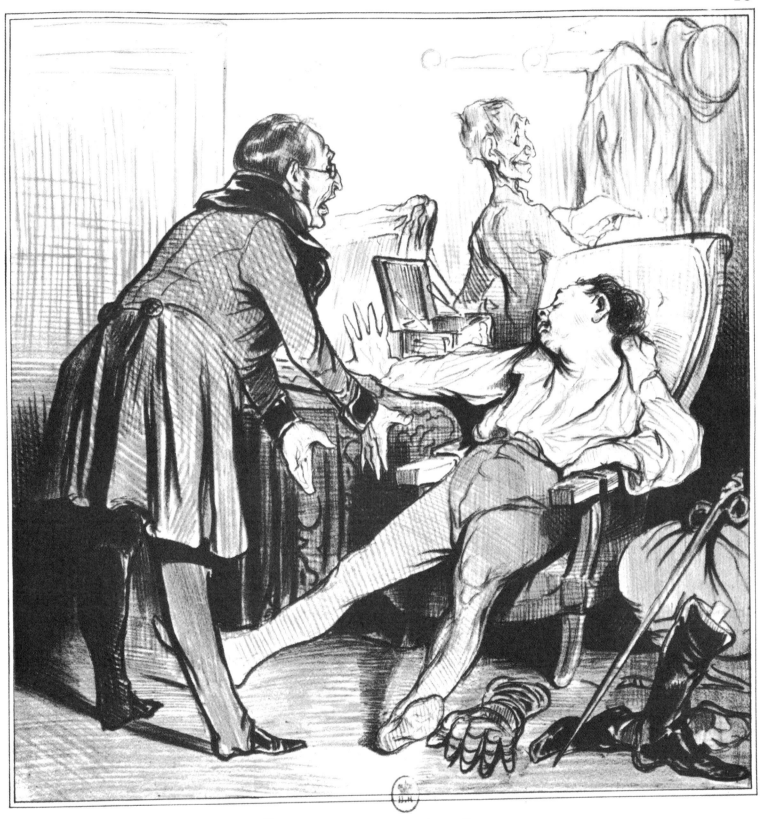

15

Recette pour guérir la colique.

Mr. Macaire, mon cher ami, ne me faites pas manquer cette soirée, j'en ai tant besoin. — Ah! mon ami, je ne puis jouer,
je souffre trop..... — Essayez, je vous en conjure...... le public vous demande il crie, menace, veut briser les banquettes,
je vais être forcé de rendre l'argent...... voyons je doublerai vos feux...... — Oh là! Oh là!..... chauffer des
serviettes!..... du vin chaud!..... chauffer, chauffer!!.... — Je triplerai vos feux.... — Chauffer toujours, chauffer!
..... chauffer les serviettes..... — Nous partagerons la recette...... — Nous partagerons la recette? levez
le rideau, la farce est jouée, le drame commence........

No. 16.   *The Beginners*

« *Bertrand — Oh no, the patient is weak, she wouldn't survive : the operation is impracticable...   Robert Macaire — Impracticable!!!   Nothing is impracticable for a beginner.   Listen, we have no name yet among the profession.   If we fail, we don't lose anything.   If, by chance we succeed... well, we'll be launched, our reputation will be made.   Both — Let's go ahead then.* »

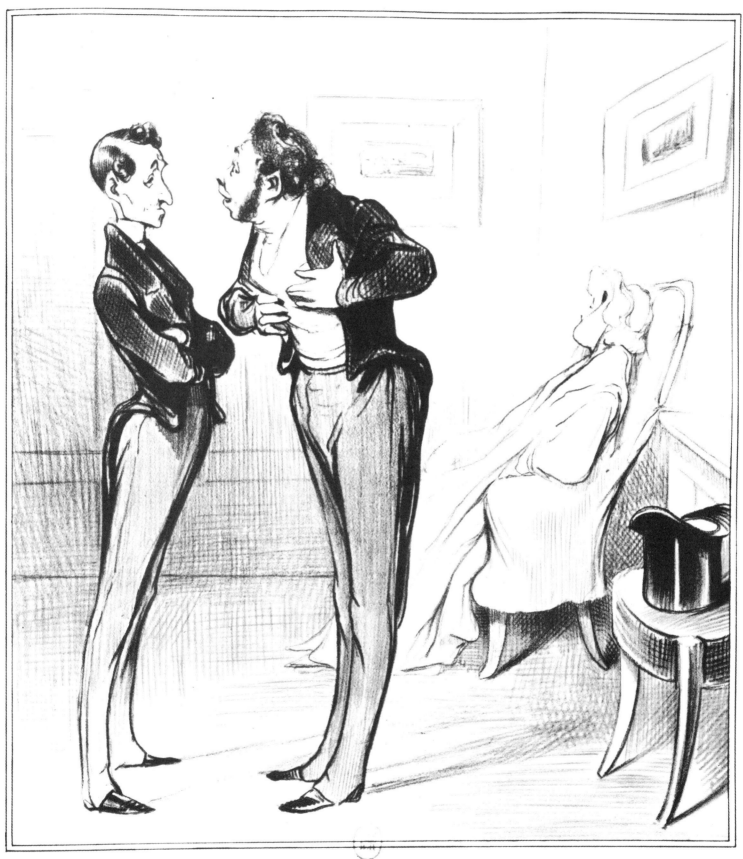

16

Le Début.

(Bertrand) Oh! non la malade est faible, elle succomberait . . . . l'opération devient impraticable . . . .
(Rob: Mac.) Impraticable!!!! . . . il n'y a rien d'impraticable pour un débutant . . . Écoute! nous sommes inconnus. Si nous
échouons, nous restons dans l'obscurité; ça ne nous recule pas. Si par hasard nous réussissons . . . . C'est fini, nous
sommes lancés, notre réputation est faite!! . . (Ensemble) Pratiquons! pratiquons.

(Donnez donc votre pratique à ces gaillards là.

No. 17. *Robert Macaire, the hypnotizer*

«*Here is an excellent subject for hypnotism. There is absolutely no connivance; I don't even know Mademoiselle de St. Bertrand, and you are going to see, gentlemen, the effect of somnambulism...*» (*Mlle. de St. Bertrand gives, in her sleep, consultations on one's illnesses, tells where treasures are hidden in the ground, advises buying stock in the Mozart Paper Co., in gold mines, or in a number of other fine enterprise.*)

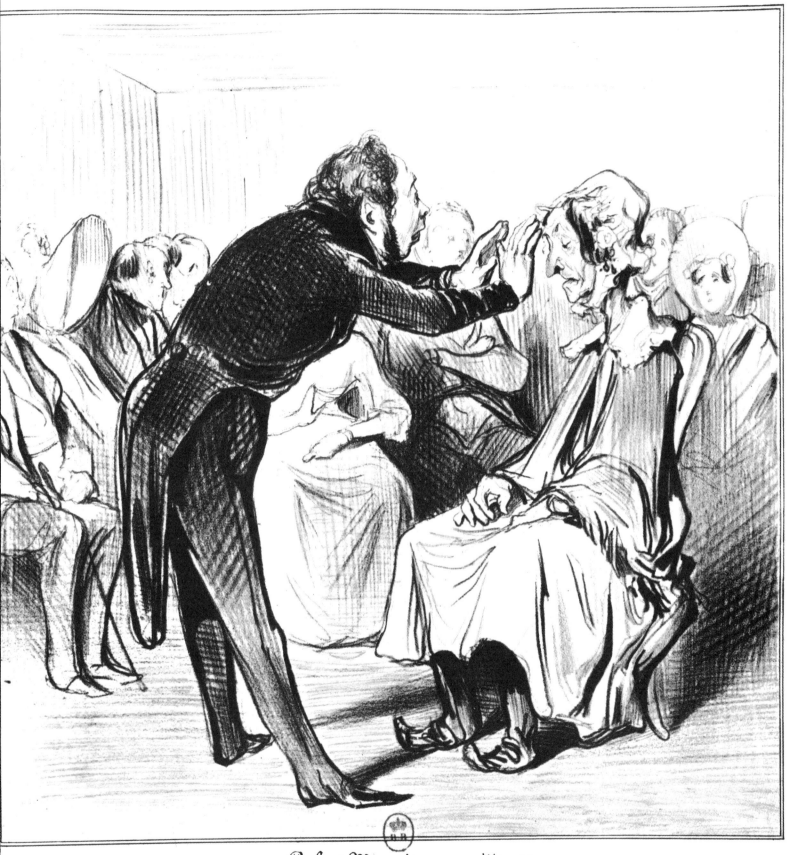

Robert Macaire magnétiseur.

Voici un excellent sujet........ pour le magnétisme........ Certes! il n'y a pas de commérage, je n'ai pas l'honneur
de connaître M.ᵉˡˡᵉ de S.ᵗᵉ Bertrand et vous allez voir Messieurs, l'effet du somnambulisme.
(M.ᵉˡˡᵉ de S.ᵗᵉ Bertrand donne dans son sommeil des consultations sur les maladies de chacun, indique des trésors
cachés sous terre, conseille de prendre des actions dans le papier Mozart, dans les mines d'or et dans une foule
d'autres fort belles opérations.)

No. 18.

«Don't talk, I hab such a co'd in by head that I can't see straight, by dear!...»

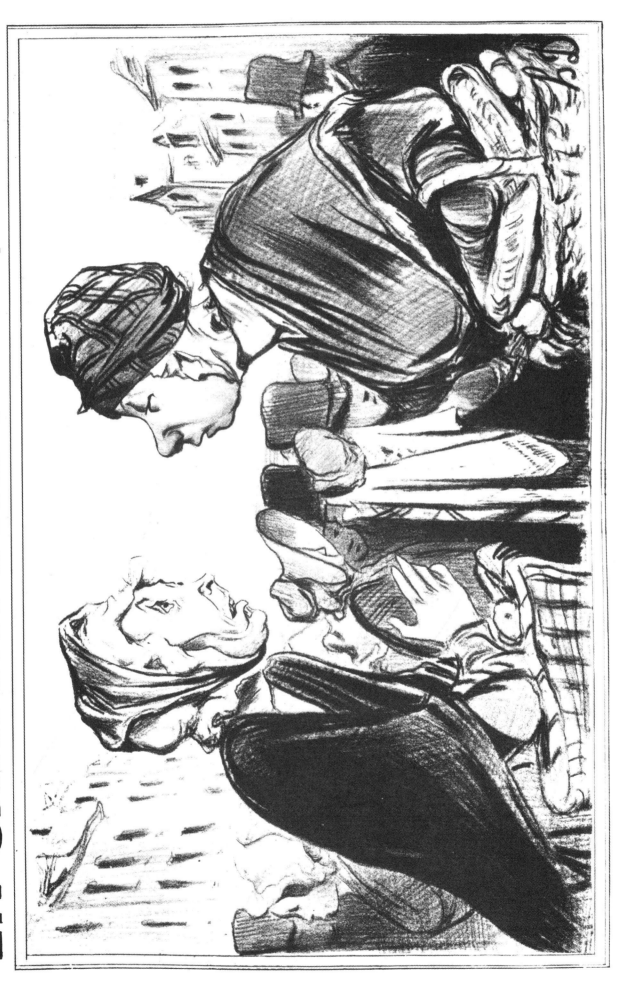

LA CARICATURE PROVISOIRE

B'en parlez pas j'suis enrubé du cerbeaux que je n'bois pas clair ma chère!.....

No. 19.
Cravings of a pregnant woman.

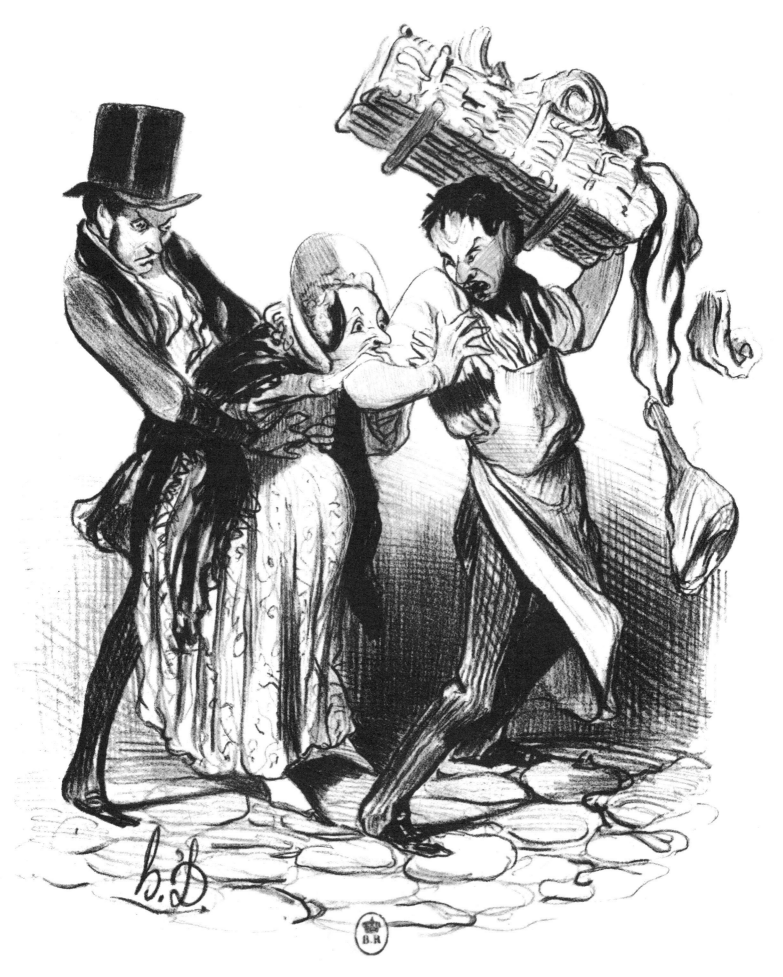

Une envie de femme grosse.

No. 20.

« The Master is ill and will receive nobody ».

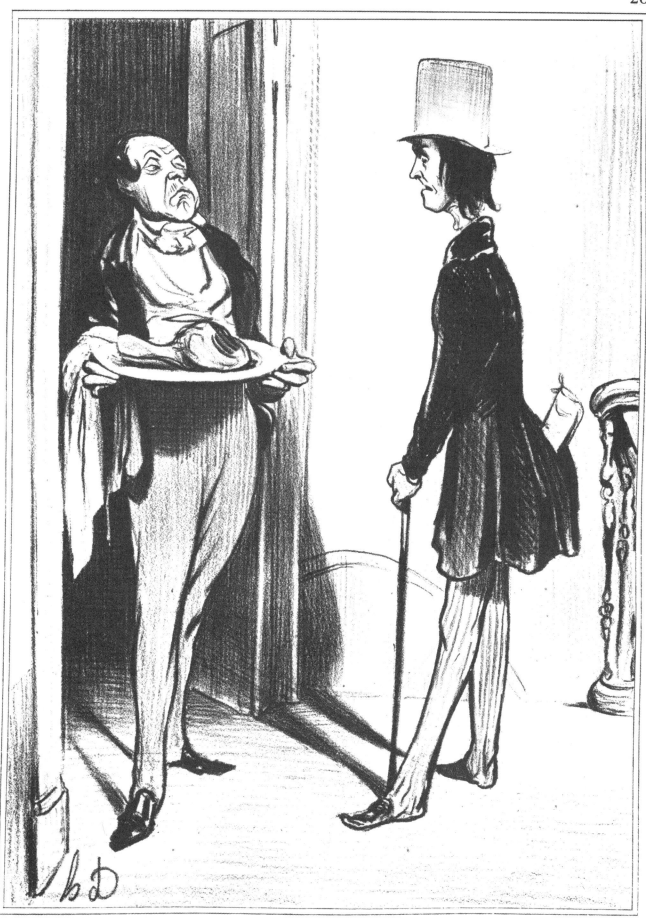

Monsieur est malade il ne recoit personne.

No. 21. *The Doctor and the Nurse*

«*How is the patient? — Alas, he died this morning at 6 o'clock. — Ah, then he didn't take my medicine. — But he did, sir. — Then he must have taken too much. — No, Doctor. — Then, he didn't take enough of it.*»

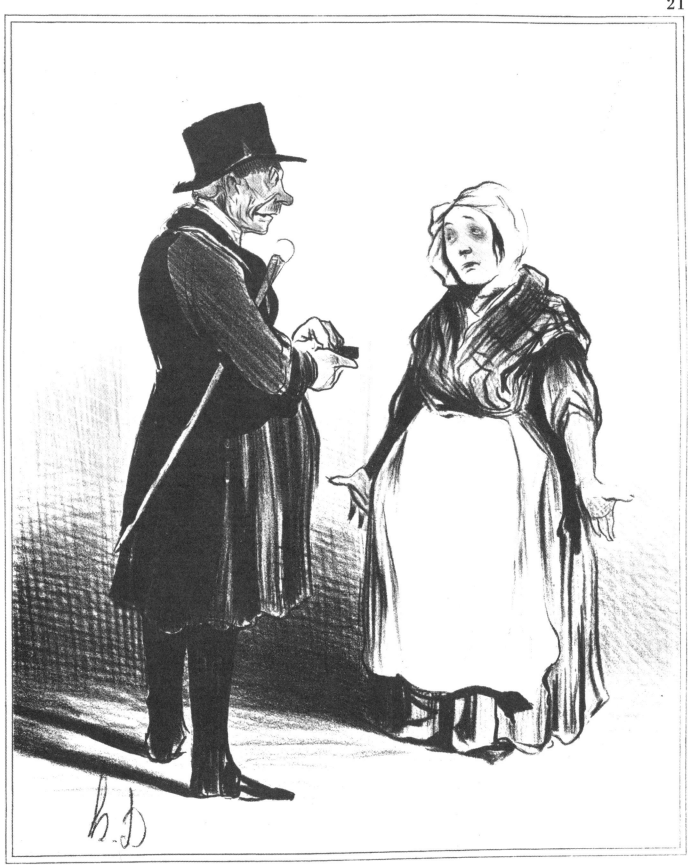

LE MÉDECIN ET LA GARDE MALADE.

Comment va le malade? Hélas Monsieur, il est mort ce matin à 6 heures! Ah! il n'a donc pas pris ma potion. — Si Monsieur. — Il en a donc trop pris. — Non Monsieur — c'est qu'il n'en a pas assez pris.

No. 22

It certainly was solid!

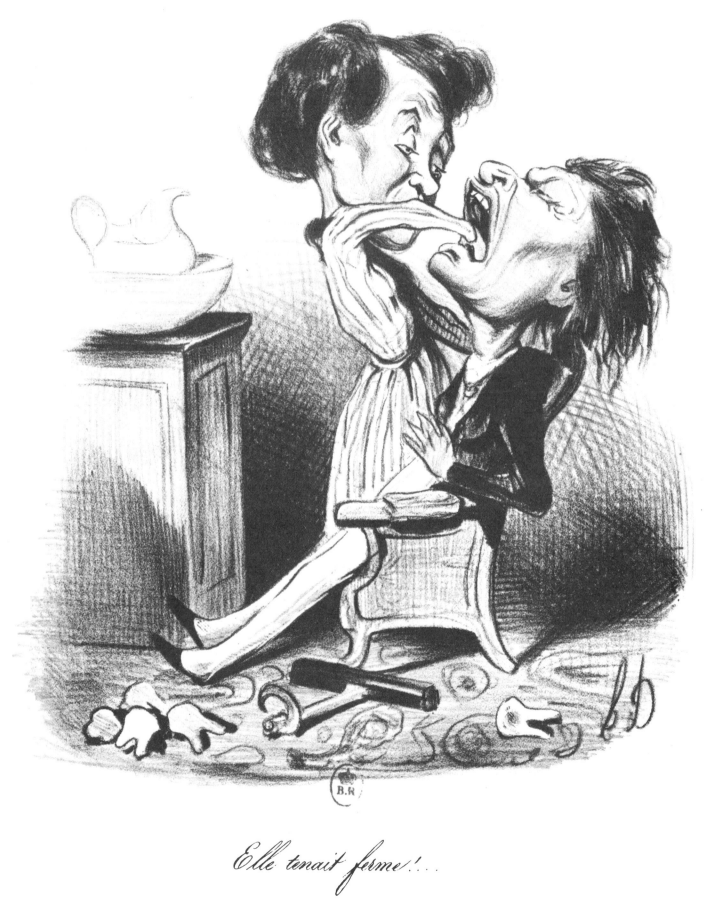

Elle tenait ferme !...

No. 23.   *The Nurse*

«No doubt about it, fruit venders are the only ones who introduce you to interesting people. An epilectic, a hydrophobic and a lunatic!... And in addition, if the grocer can get me that tuberculosis he promised me, that would be darned nice for me.»

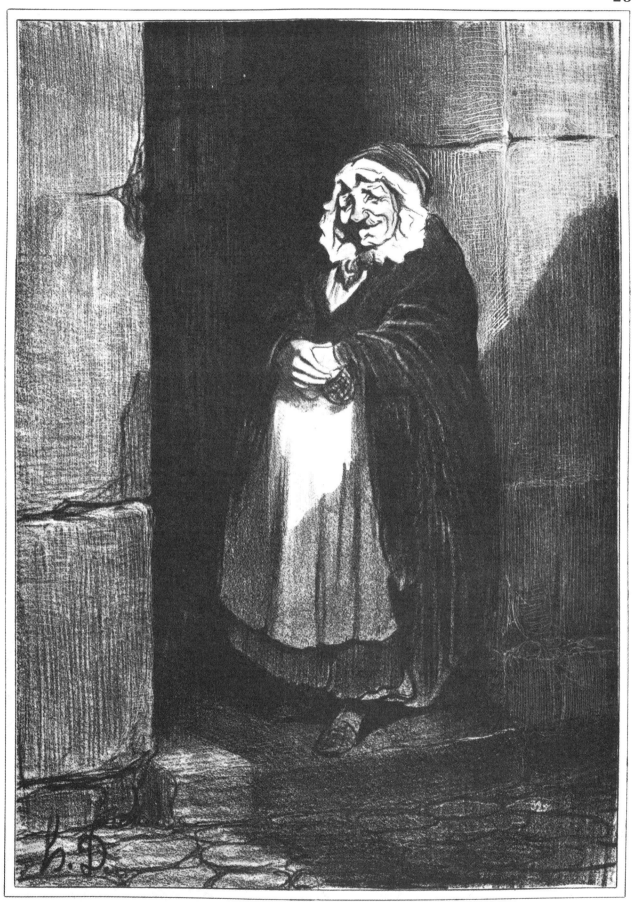

LA GARDE-MALADE.

Décidément, il n'y a que les fruitières pour vous procurer de belles connaissances . Un épileptique, un hydrophobe et une folle !...... Si l'épicier pouvait me faire avoir avec cà la maladie de poitrine qu'il m'a promise, c'est ca qui me ferait joliment du bien !

No. 24.   *The. Hypochondriac*

This category of citizen is the providence of the medical profession, the benediction of the drug trade. It is the nymph Egeria whose inspiration was responsible for white mustard, red Paraguay, Regnault paste, the Clyso-bol, and in general all inventions for relieving unsuffering humanity. The hypochondriac is the prey, one after the other of pleurisy, consumption and so forth and so forth... He varies his ills in order to vary his pleasures and every day he exclaims when he feels his pulse : «Really, my health must be good and sound to be able to resist all these diseases.»

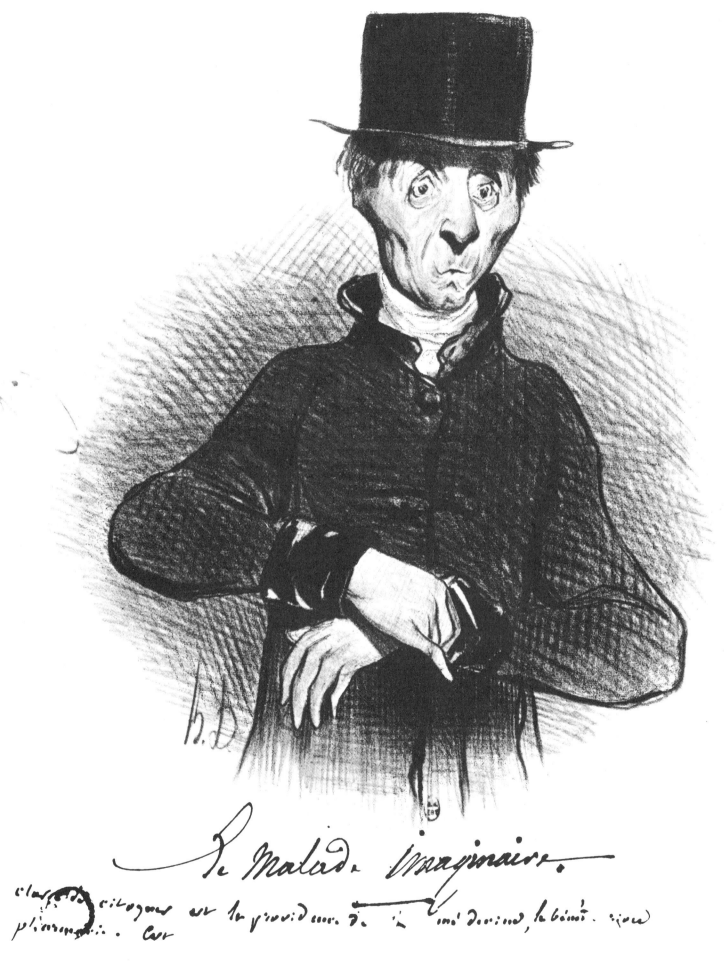

Le Malade imaginaire.

No. 25.   *The Squint*

«*Lord! I didn't recognize you! — Oh, that's because I had an operation. I'm no longer cross-eyed, and that changes my looks completely, don't you think so? — Yes, completely. Before, you squinted toward the outside...*»

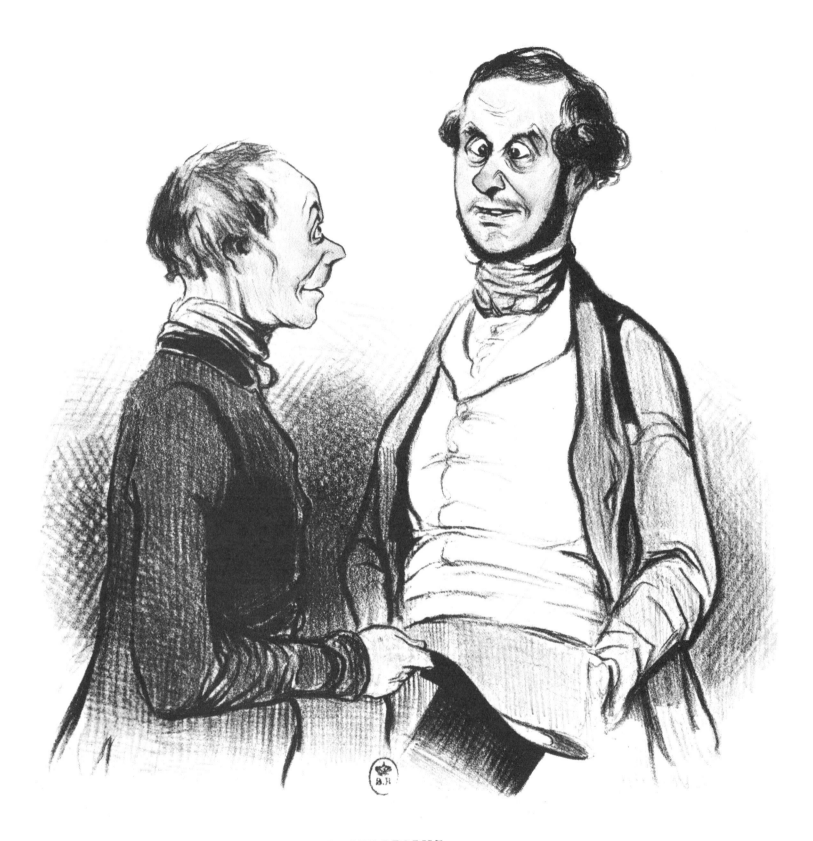

LE STRABISME,

—Ma foi je ne vous reconnaissais pas !—Ah! c'est que je me suis fait opérer, je ne louche plus ca me change tout-
à-fait n'est-ce-pas!—Oh! tout-à-fait, car avant vous louchiez en dehors je crois . . . .

No. 26.   *The Hydropathic Doctor*

«Today, two bucketsful will do... tomorrow you can bring four. — Ah, what a fine doctor!... One can't like water too much... (aside) I'm only afraid it'll end up by killing his taste for food forever!...»

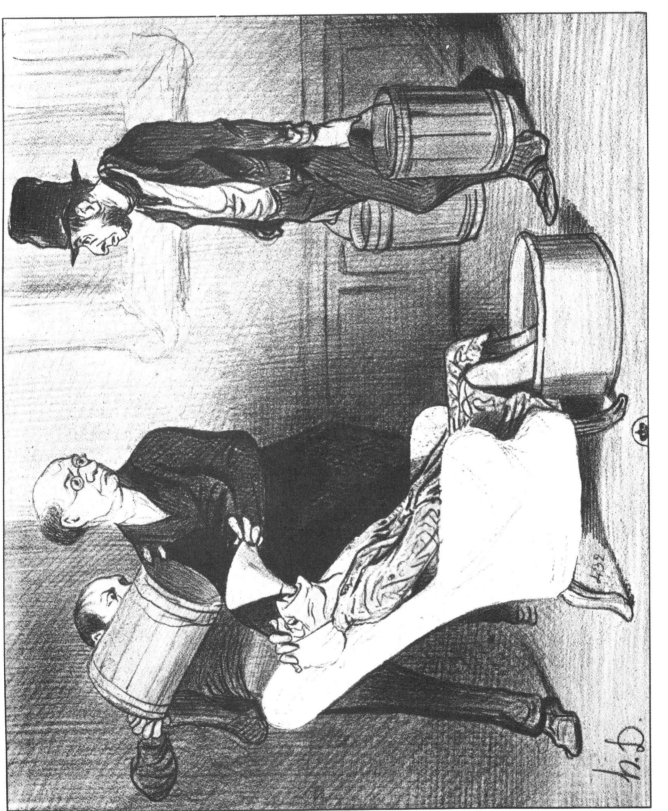

LE MÉDECIN HYDROPATHE.

– Aujourd'hui nous nous contenterons de deux voies.... demain vous m'en apporterez quatre voies........
– Ah! ché cha un bon medechin !..... on ne chaurait jamais trop donner le ſout de l'eau.....(à part) je crains seulement
que cha ne lui fasse pacher le ſout du pain !.....

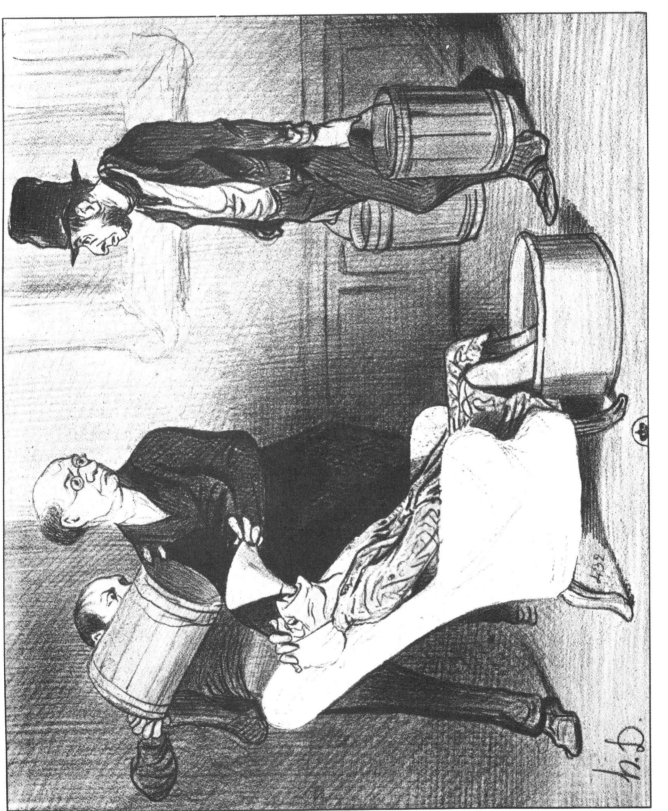

No. 27. *A Lucky Find*

«*By Jove, I'm delighted! You have yellow fever... it will be the first time I've been lucky enough to treat this disease!*»

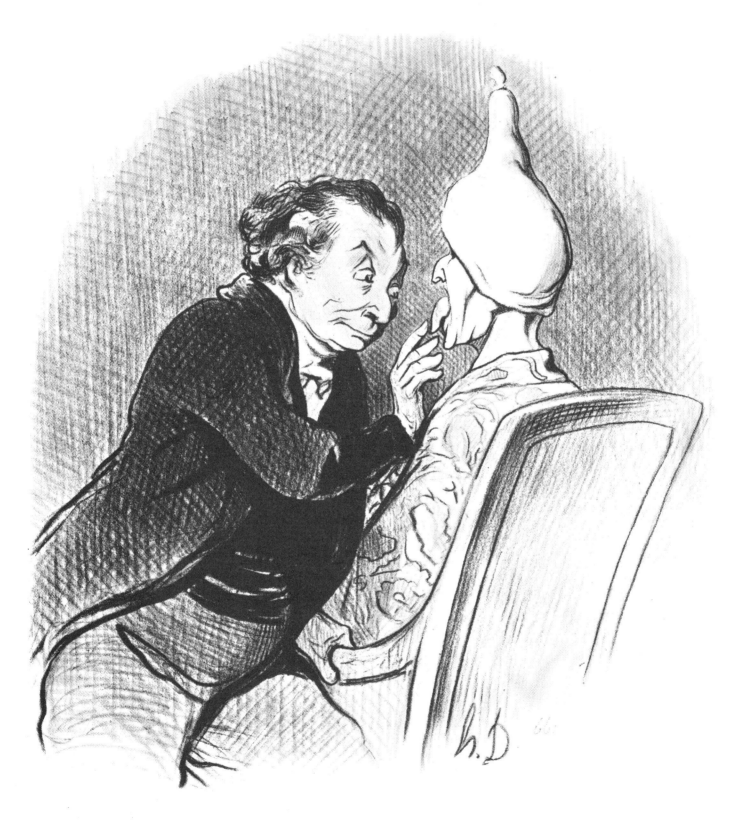

UNE HEUREUSE TROUVAILLE.

Parbleu je suis ravi.....vous avez la fièvre jaune.....c'est la première fois de ma vie que j'ai le bonheur d'en soigner une !

No. 28. *Camphor cigarettes*

«I've been told they're wonderful for putting on weight!... — And I've been assured that they're infallible for reducing!...»

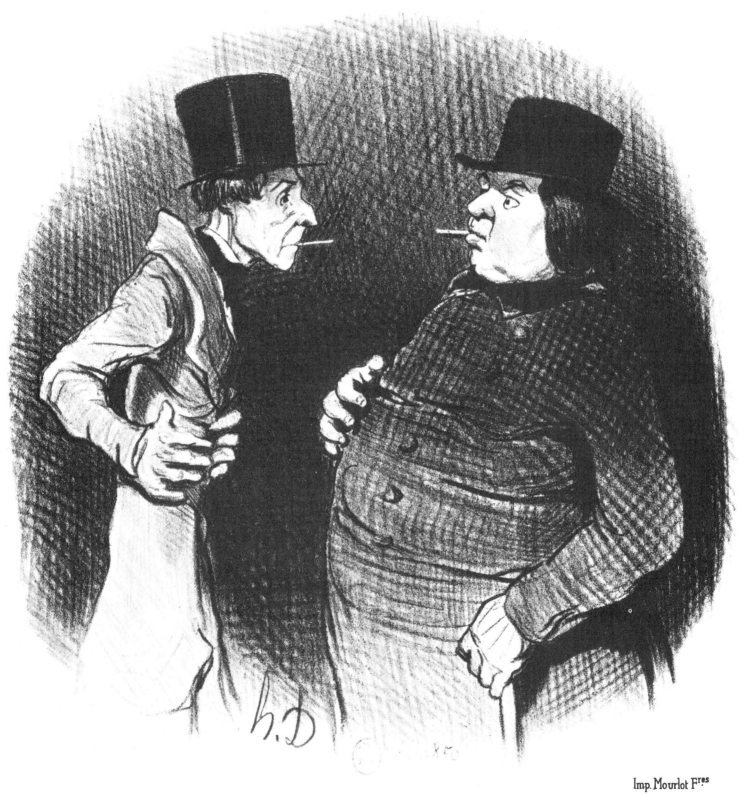

Imp. Mourlot F^{res}

LES CIGARETTES DE CAMPHRE.

— On m'a certifié que c'était excellent pour engraisser !..
— On m'a juré que c'était souverain pour faire maigrir !..

No. 29.

«Look at this fool who does not even notice that his barrell is leaking... — You're ignorant! It is on purpose, it's chloride which is being sprayed on the streets to disinfect them... it's the Labaraque *system, applied to the city of Paris.»*

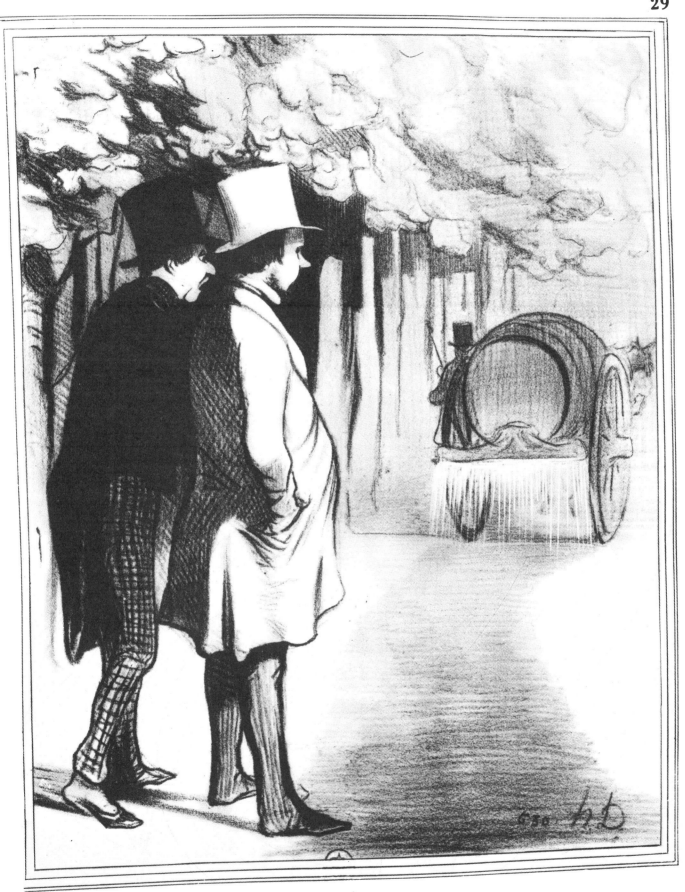

— Vois-tu cet imbécile qui ne s'apperçoit pas que son tonneau fuit......
— T'es bête ! c'est fait exprès, c'est du chlorure qu'on répand dans les rues pour les désinfecter
c'est le système **Labaraque**, appliqué à la ville de Paris.

No. 30.

Yesterday in the Rue Saint-Honoré, a dignified elderly man was felled by an attack of apoplexy. It would have been the end of him if by chance the well known Dr. Cabassol who happened to be at his window at No. 107, had not hastened to his help. Thanks to his intelligent treatment and devoted care, the patient was quickly revived. Our famous Dr. Cabassol, adding to his generous attentions, refused to accept any payment other than the thanks of a family that will eternally bless his name. Glory to Dr. Cabassol. — «You know, you're the one who was the dignified old man. You might have fallen on your way to see me yesterday, you might have hurt yourself, and then I could have come to your help. I have presented all this in a more dramatic way for the newspapers. It won't do you any harm and it'll do me a lot of good!...»

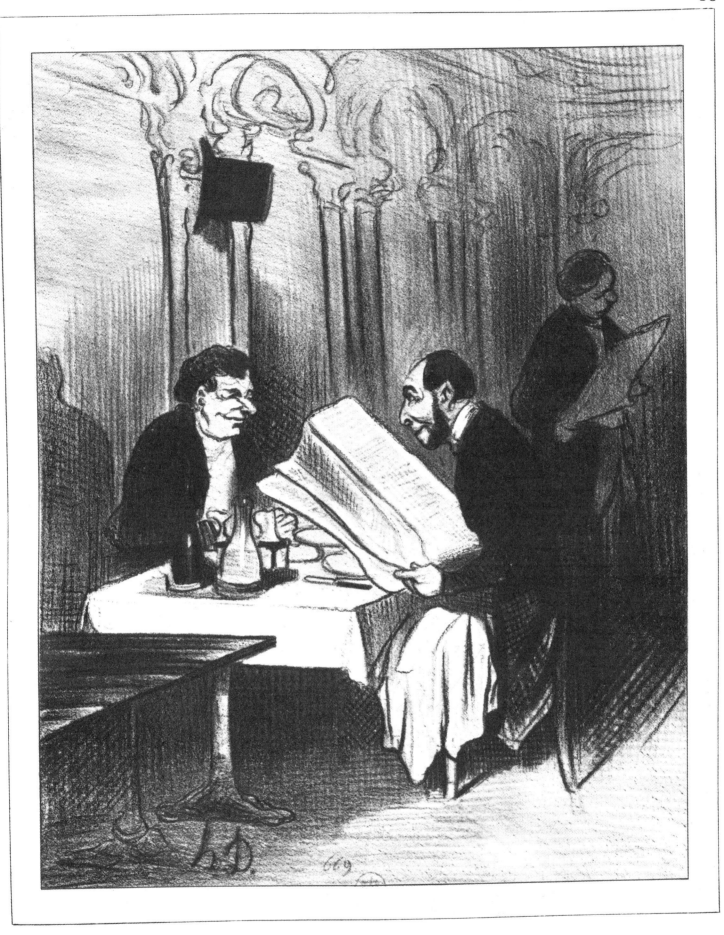

« hier, dans la rue St Honoré, un respectable vieillard, tombât frappé d'une attaque d'appoplexie, c'en était fait de lui si par hasard le célèbre docteur Cabassol qui était à sa fenêtre au N°107, ne s'était empressé de voler à son secours, grâce à des soins intelligens et prodigués avec la plus touchante sollicitude, le malade fut promptement rappelé à la vie. Notre célèbre docteur Cabassol mettant le comble à sa généreuse conduite n'a voulu recevoir pour récompense de ses soins que les remerciemens d'une famille qui bénira éternellement son nom. Honneur au docteur Cabassol! »

—Dites donc, c'est vous le respectable vieillard en question, hier vous avez manqué de tomber en venant me voir, vous auriez pu vous blesser et alors j'aurais pu vous secourir... j'ai arrangé tout ça d'une manière un peu plus dramatique pour le journal... ça ne vous fait pas de mal et ça me fera grand bien!

No. 31.

«Yes sir... dedicated by my profession and my sentiments to the purest philanthropy, I have not hesitated to spend my nights nor to use up my retorts and stills, to discover a salve more Regnauld (Regnauld was the name of a popular salve) than anything known to this day... I have finally realized my dreams... that is to say, the fusion of wood lice and slugs... as my first care is to relieve suffering and coughing humanity, in spite of the high price of the raw materials, I sell the box for only five francs... half a box cured Mr. Ducantal senior...»

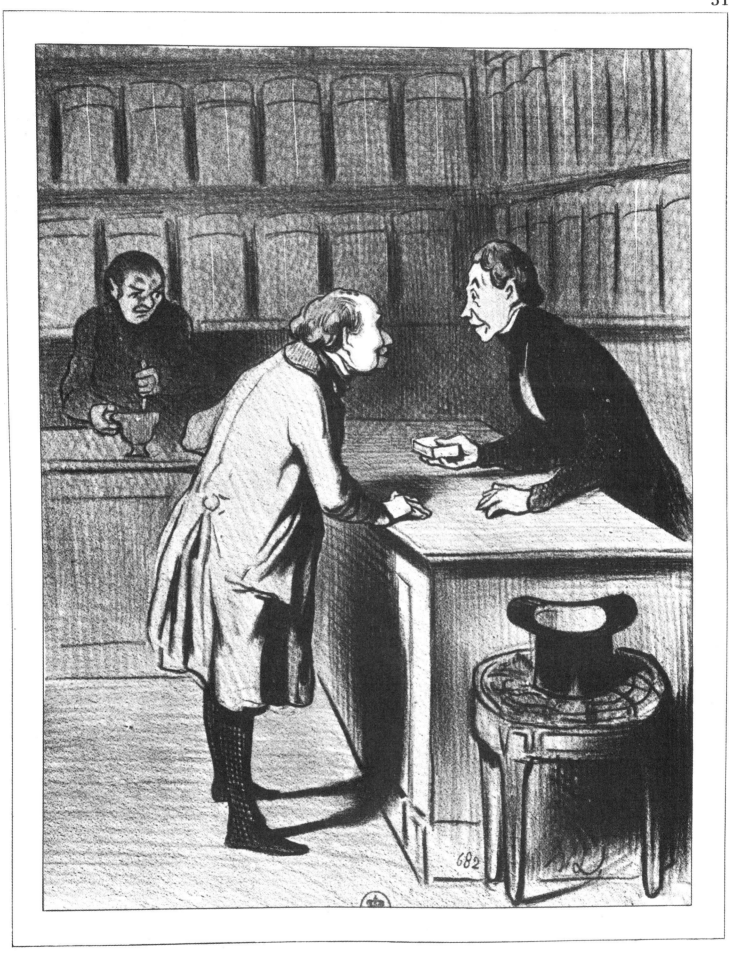

Oui monsieur.... dévoué par état et par sentiment à la philantropie la plus pure, je n'ai reculé devant aucunes veilles ni aucunes cornues pour arriver à trouver une pâte encore plus Regnauld que tout ce qui s'est fait jusqu'à ce jour...je suis enfin arrivé au but de mes rêves....c'est à dire à la fusion du cloporte au limaçon.... comme avant tout je ne veux que le soulagement de l'humanité souffrante et toussante, malgré le haut prix des matières premières je ne vends la boîte que cinq francs....une demi-boite a suffi pour guérir M.r Ducantal père!..

No. 32.

«My dear fellow, I give you my word that you look very ill this morning. I'm talking not as your doctor but as your friend, I insist on treating you... better than I would myself. I'm going to apply thirty leeches to your epigastrium and if tomorrow I don't find you improved, I'll apply sixty...»

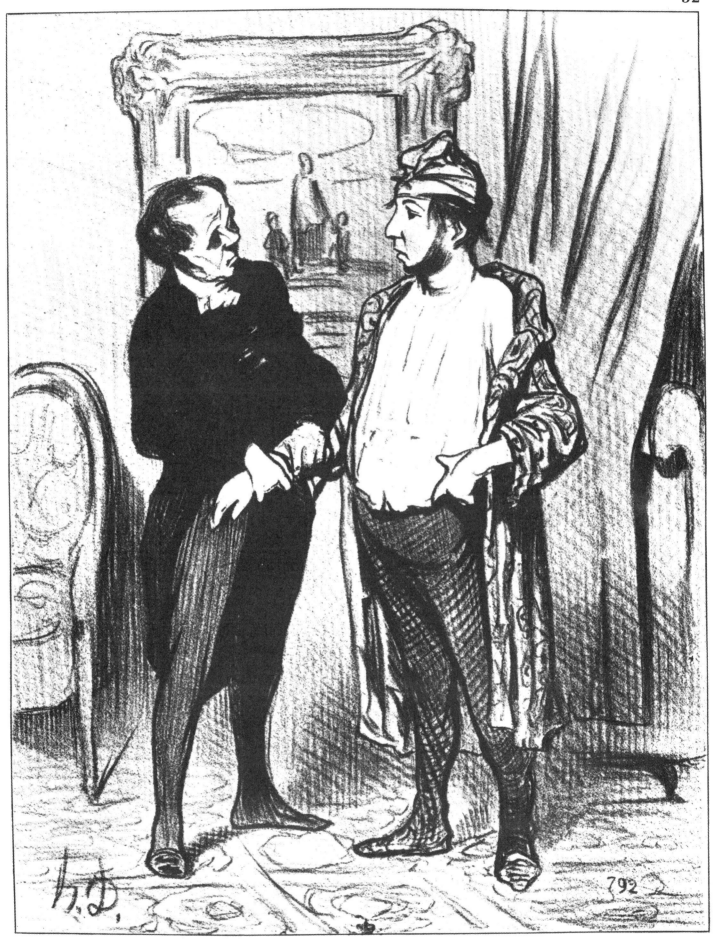

—Mon cher je t'assure que je te trouve mauvaise mine ce matin.... ce n'est pas en médecin que je te parle, c'est en ami.... je veux absolument te soigner.... mieux que je ne me soignerais moi-même..... je vais t'appliquer trente sangsues à l'épigastre, et si demain matin je ne te trouve pas plus robuste, je t'en réappliquerai soixante!.....

No. 33.

«Ouch!... Ouch!... — Fine... fine... that proves it's coming!...»

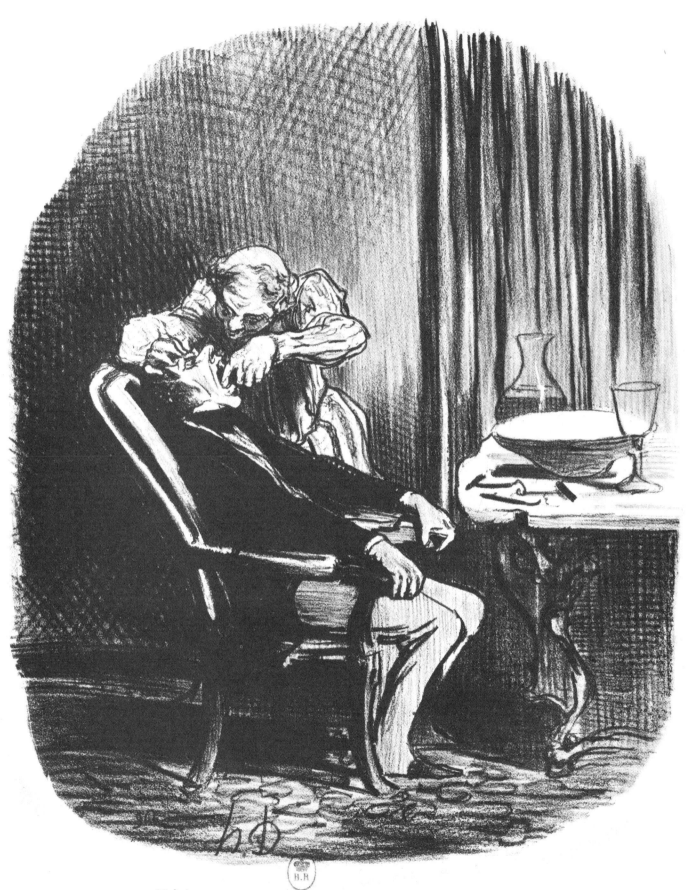

—Oh! la ... . la ... . la ... . . la!
—Tant mieux ... . tant mieux ... . . . ça prouve qu'elle vient! ...

No. 34.

«Doctor, I believe I'm consumptive.»

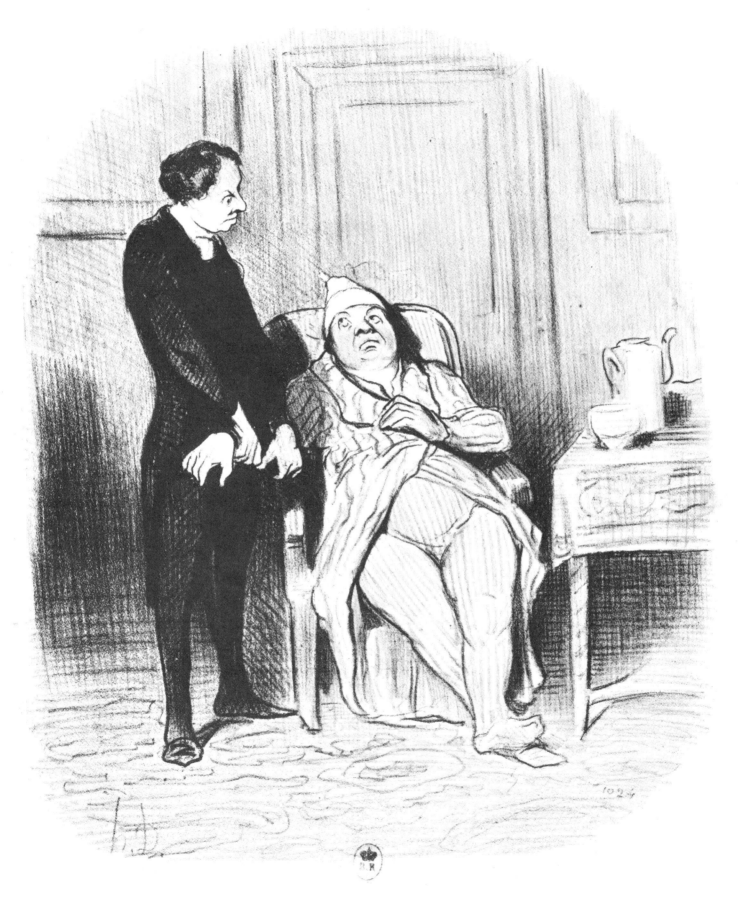

— Ah! docteur.... je crois bien que j'suis poitrinaire!....

No. 35.

« The patient — What, doctor! Not even a soft boiled egg! The doctor — «No, you'll have to keep to the strictest diet for five more days... It's a mistake to think we must eat to live!... Excuse me if I run along, I have a dinner engagement!...»

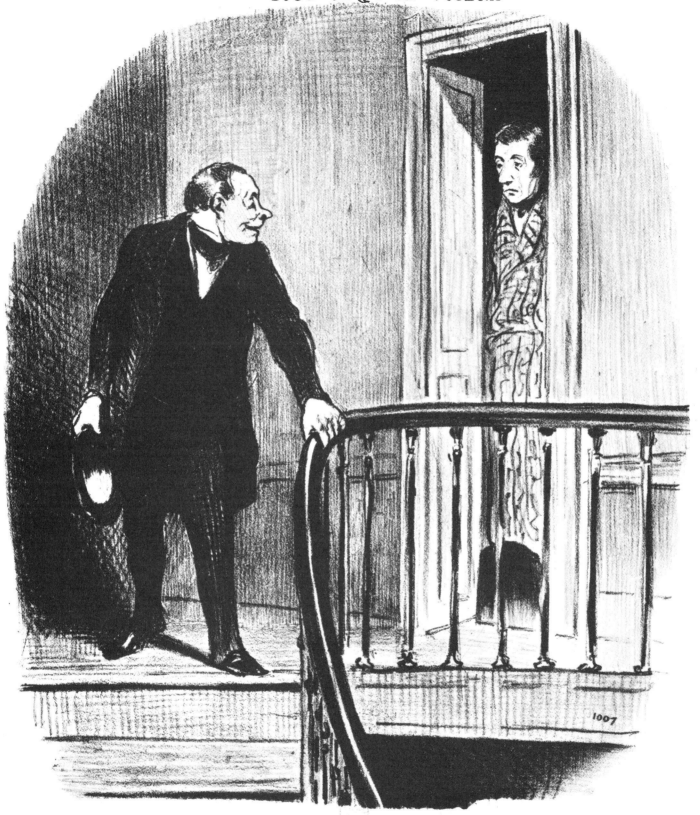

Le malade.—Comment, docteur, pas même un œuf à la coque!

Le docteur.—Non; il faut que vous observiez la diète la plus complète pendant encore au moins cinq jours... c'est un préjugé de croire qu'on a besoin de manger pour vivre!.. Pardon si je vous quitte si vite, je vais diner en ville!..

No. 36.

Doctor Véron having renounced politics, its pomp and its works, retires to the country, at Auteuil and devotes himself to the favorite pastimes of the Arcadian shepherds of old; the true sage consoles himself with some philosophy and clarinet.

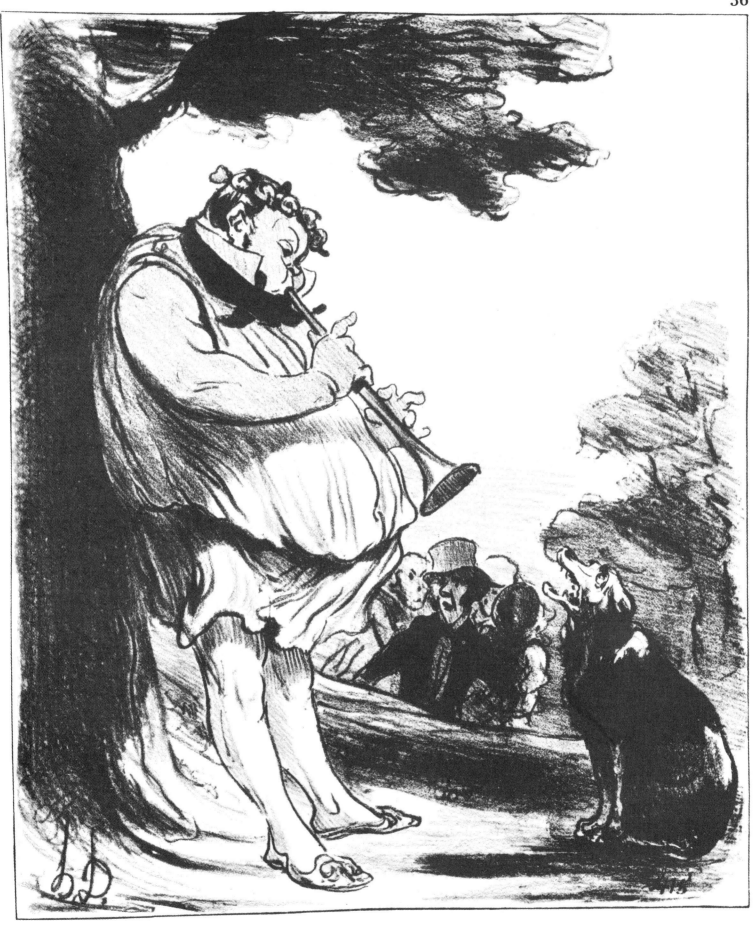

Le Docteur Véron ayant renoncé à la politique à ses pompes et à ses œuvres se retire à la campagne à Auteuil, et s'y livre aux divertissemens favoris des anciens bergers de l'Arcadie : le vrai sage se console de tout avec de la Philosophie et une clarinette.

No. 37.   *The Grippe Epidemic in Paris*

«How are you coughing? — I'm coughing quite well, thank you,... and you?»

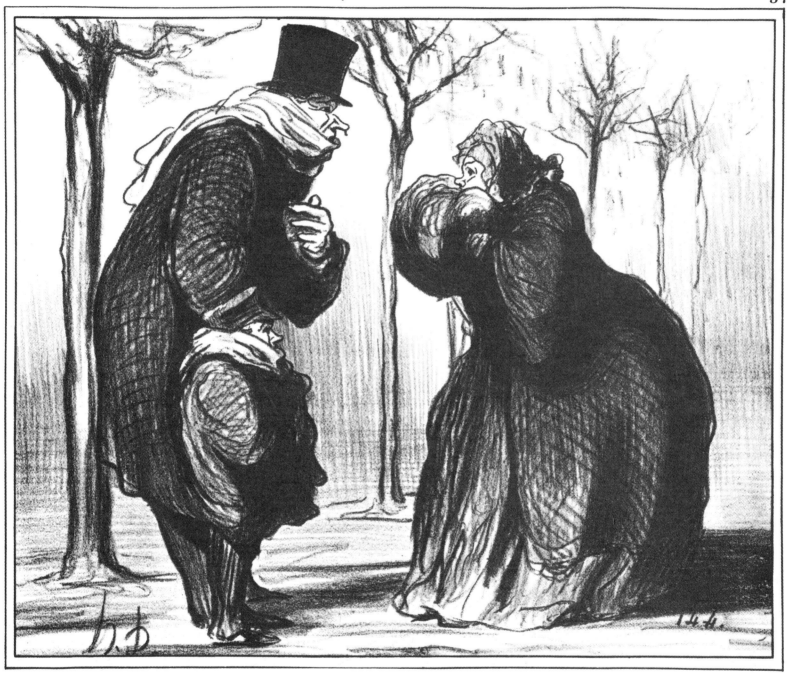

PARIS GRIPPÉ.

_ Comment toussez-vous ?......
_ Vous êtes bien bonne..., je tousse assez bien...... et vous ?....

No. 38.

«Come along, dear, I don't think that picture pretty. — Oh! yes, it is... as a pharmacist it interests me greatly.
The picture certainly represents the testing of a new medicine... let's see what the catalogue says?...»

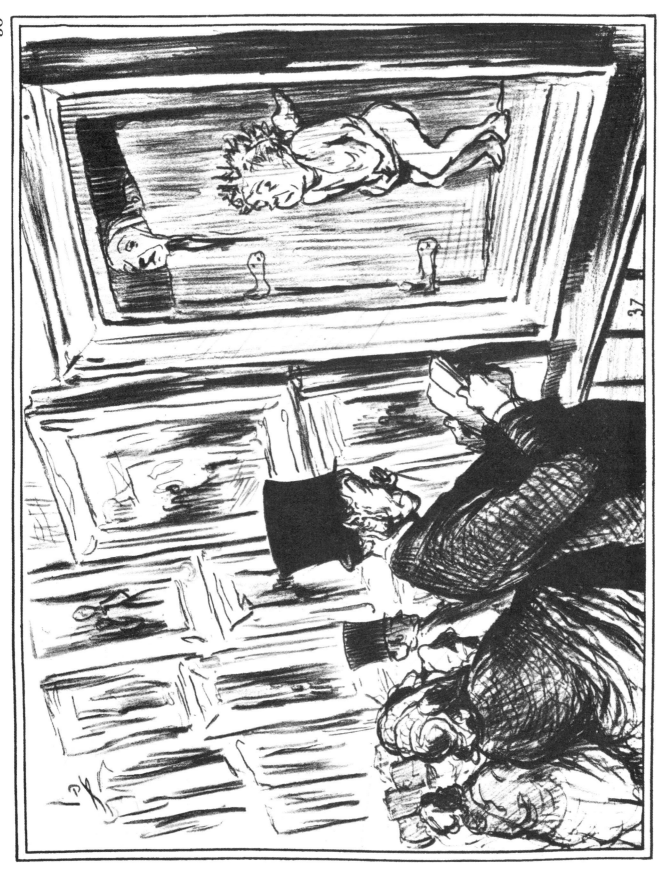

— Viens donc..., mon ami, je ne trouve pas ce tableau joli.

— Si fait, en ma qualité de pharmacien, il m'intéresse beaucoup ...ce tableau représente sans doute, l'essai d'une nouvelle médecine.... voyons ce que dit mon livret ?.......

No. 39.

Esculapius, prepared to defend energetically his position against all innovators (blond or dark), who come to attack it.

ACTUALITES.

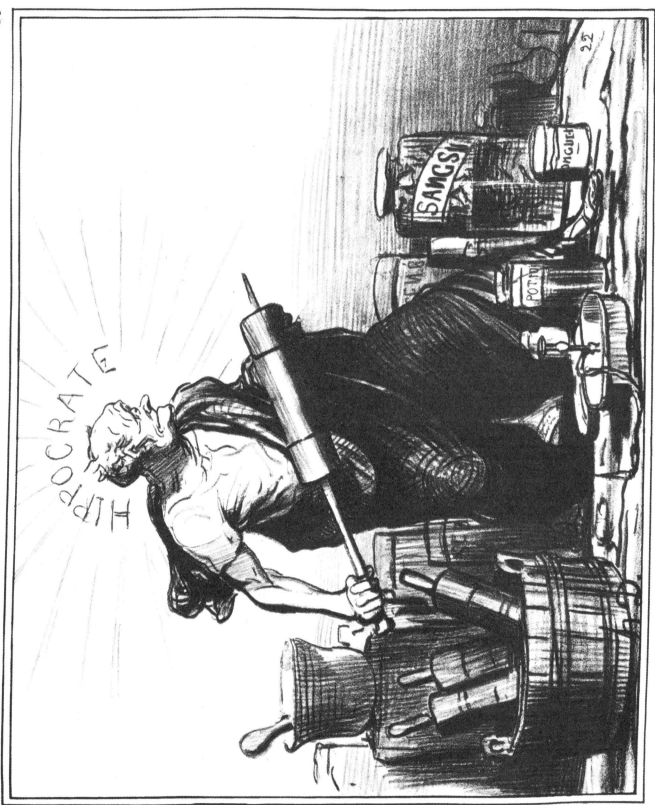

Esculape se mettant en garde pour défendre énergiquement sa position, contre tous les novateurs blonds
en noirs, qui viennent pour l'attaquer !......

No. 40.

Paris in the throes of the grippe.

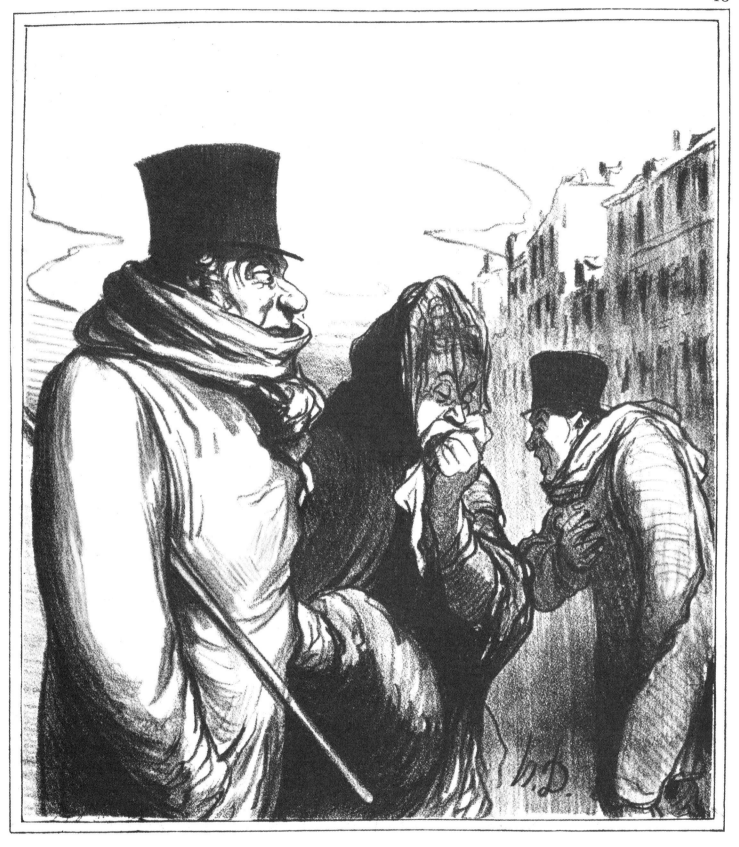

Paris grippé

No. 41.

«Come on... let's open our mouth.»

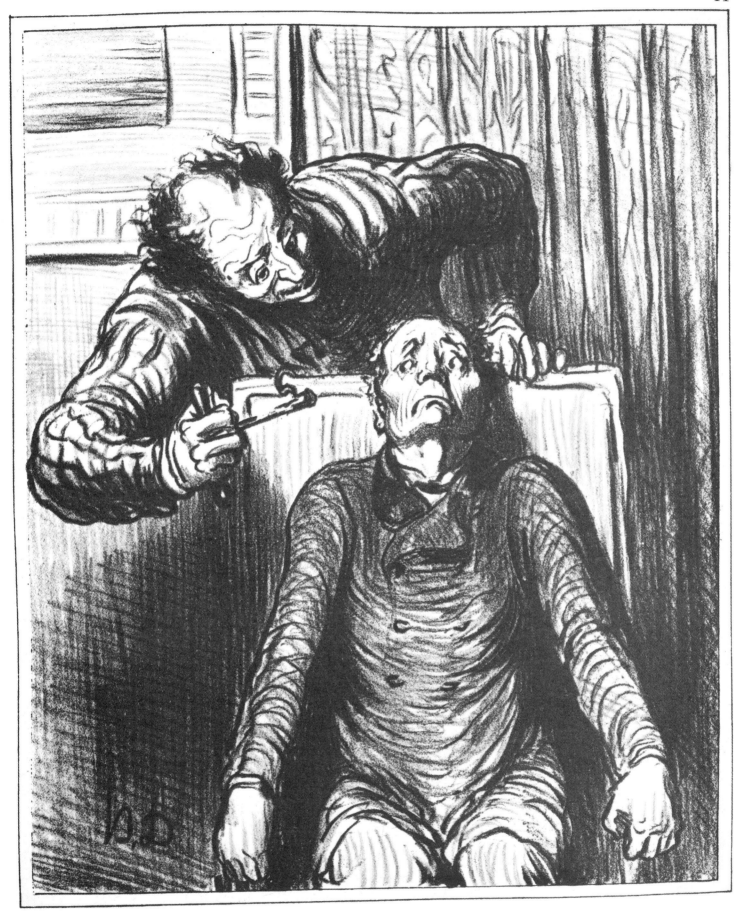

— Voyons .... ouvrons la bouche ! ....

No. 42.

«Aren't you taking anything? — No, I'm afraid. — Oh, come! a laudanum grog!»

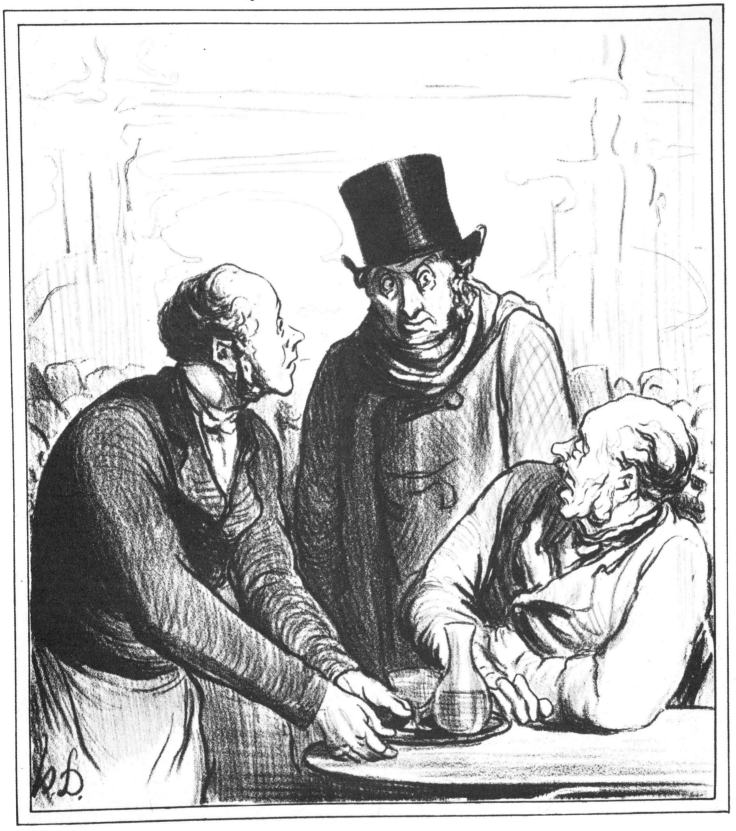

_ Vous ne prenez rien ?...
_ Non, j'ai peur....
_ Allons, un grog au laudanum !...

No. 43.

«Yesterday the breech-loading gun (aiguille refers to steel igniting pin of such a gun), tomorrow, those fellows. Will we be better off?»

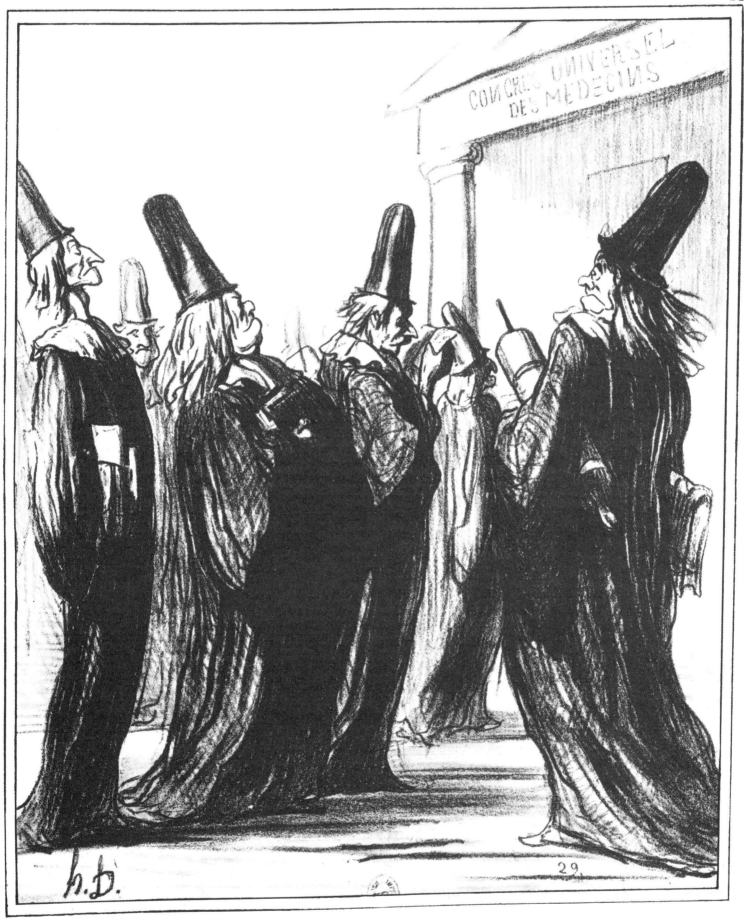

Hier le fusil à aiguille; eux demain: gagnerons-nous au change?

No. 44.

Academic Reception.

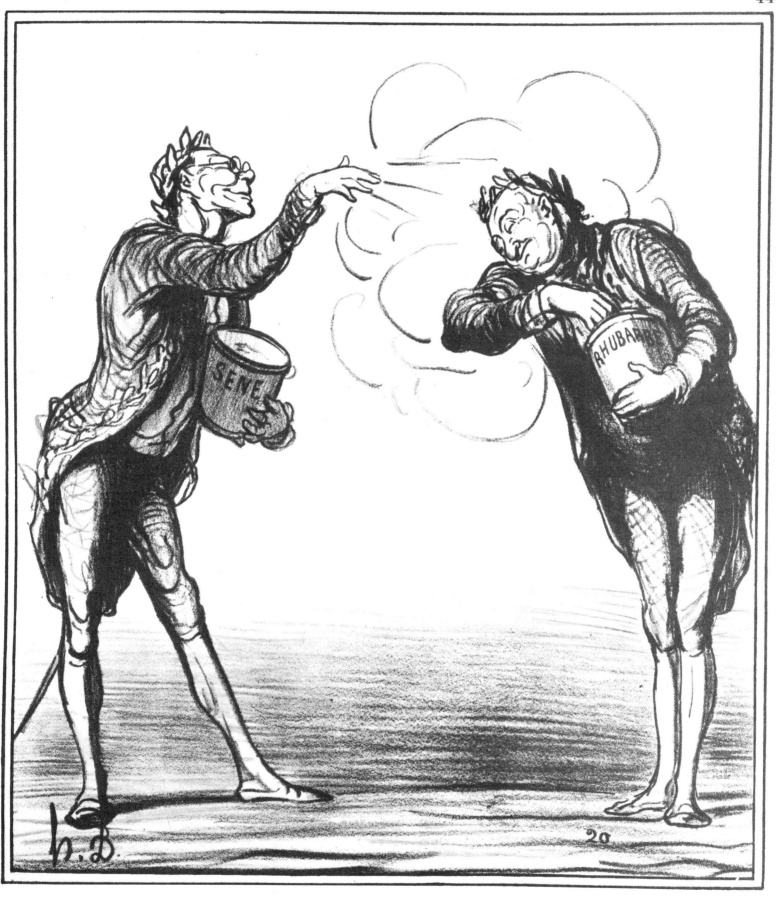

Reception académique.

No. 45. *Cramps*
«*Oh! Oh! Oh! my stomach!*»

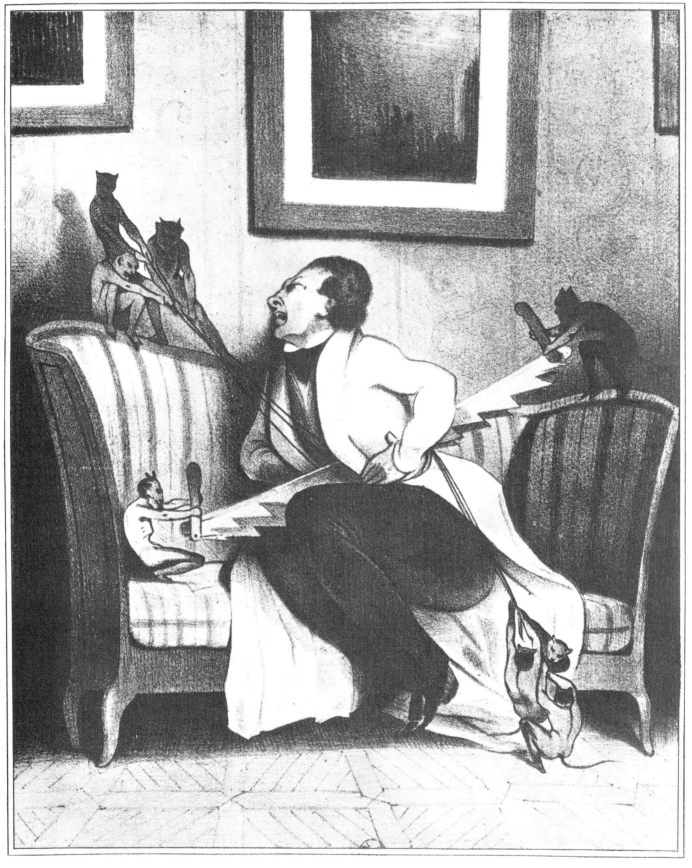

La Colique
Hola! hola!......hola! le ventre!.... hola!!

No. 46.   *The Headache*

«Oh! Oh! Bang-bang-ding-a-ling Oh!»

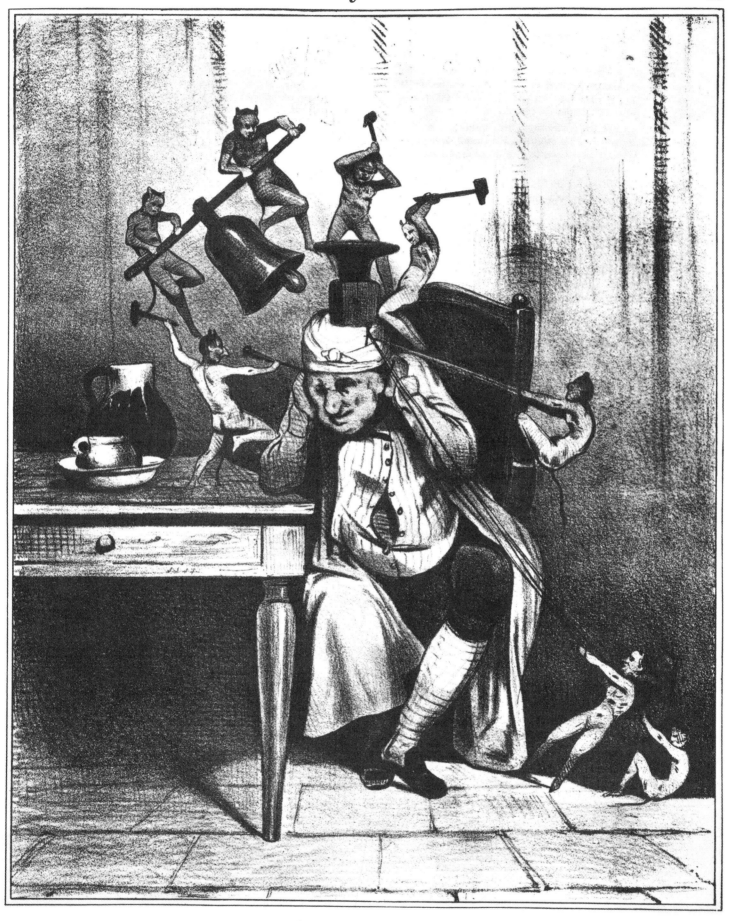

Le mal de tête.

Hola! hola! ... pan! pan! ... dindrelindin — dindrelindin hola! hola! hola!!

No. 47.   *The Hypochondriac*

«*I'm done for... I'll have to make my will... They're going to bury me... farewell.*»

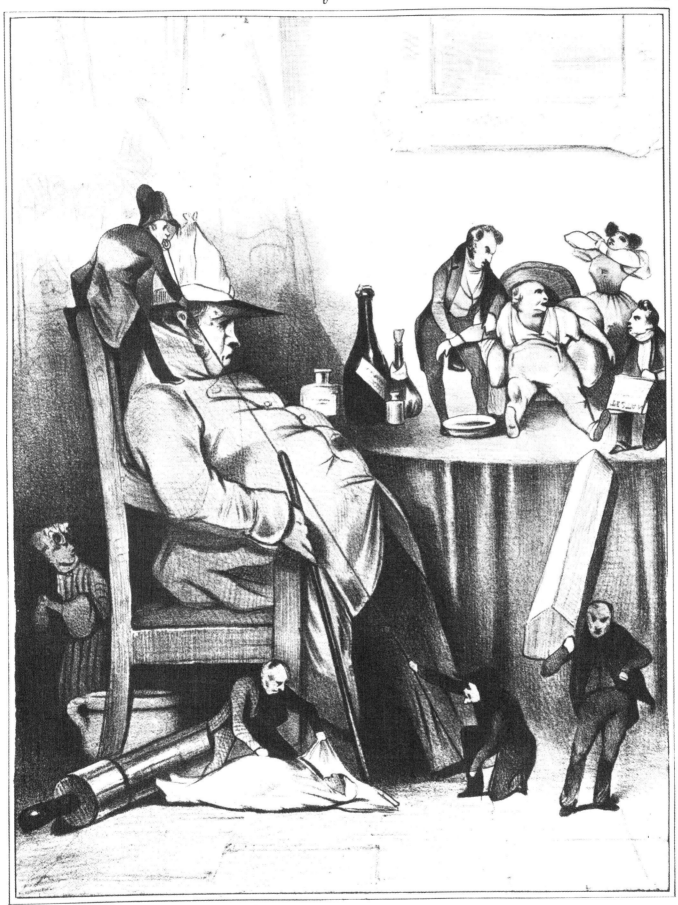

Le malade imaginaire.

Je suis perdu.... il faut faire mon testament.... ils vont m'ensevelir... m'enterrer.....
adieu !

No. 48.   *The Doctor*

*«How the devil does it happen that all my patients succumb?... Yet I bleed them, I physic them, I drug them...
I simply can't understand!»*

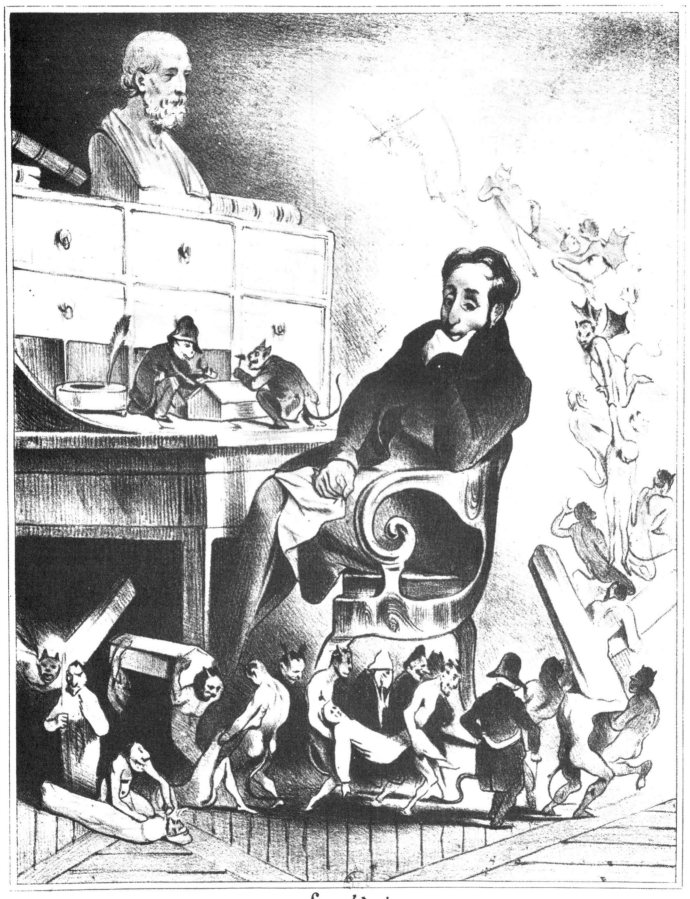

Le médecin,

Pourquoi, diable! mes malades s'en vont ils donc tous?............ j'ai beau les saigner, les purger, les droguer............ je n'y comprends rien!

*D*OCTORS *do not appear to have roused in Daumier quite such intense interest and savage irony as he reserved for lawyers. His mockery seems to have been fortuitous, at least during the first half of his life, though it became increasingly bitter and spontaneous as he grew older.*

It seems, as Professor Mondor points out, that he himself seldom needed medical advice. Daumier was of medium height and well-built, and apparently he was of strong constitution and remained for a long time in good health.

Nevertheless, there are certain details which seem to have escaped his biographers, all of whom have insisted on his robust health. First of all, he had an impediment in his speech, which he disguised by keeping a short pipe constantly in his mouth. His « pipette » was famous and provided him with an excuse for never speaking. Though the nineteenth century was fertile in witticisms he himself was never credited with uttering one, in spite of the fact that he frequented a talkative and witty circle of friends. Furthermore, he must have received a slash on the forehead from a policeman's sword in 1830, for his portrait by Feuchère, painted about 1833, shows a long scar receding into the hair. This scar is no longer visible in subsequent portraits.

At a certain period the subject of pregnant women and their fancies seems to have been familiar to him. Perhaps this period corresponded with that of his marriage, which followed the birth of a natural child, who doubtless died young and who figures under his own surname and christian name in the Registrar General's Office in Paris.

Daumier was never really ill, however, till about 1856, when he was roughly fifty years old. His exhaustion becomes visible in his lithographs but we hear of it too in a letter from Baudelaire to Le Maréchal, dated 1858 and ending with the words : « I am at Daumier's place in the Ile Saint-Louis. He has been near to death these last days and I am keeping his wife company. » Daumier's weariness, this attack of exhaustion that can be accounted for by his age, was doubtless serious but he recovered from it, since we find him starting work again about 1859-1860.

It was not till thirteen years later, in 1873, that he was forced to have recourse to a surgeon when one of his eyelids began to droop over the eye.

Perhaps the sight of this eye had been bad for a long time. His friends have mentioned the way his eyes blinked and Nadar's photographs show it clearly. In any case, his sight became so weak after 1873 that his doctor forbade him to work and in 1878, just at the time of the individual exhibition which his friends considered as a revenge and a revelation, he was kept at home by a recent operation for cataract. In the winter of this year of 1878, he had a stroke from which he never recovered and he died shortly after, in 1879.

It would be interesting, if this were not rendered impossible by the inadequacy of the available information and the scarcity of documents, to consider certain other questions. Daumier, who, as Professor Mondor remarks, was not deeply interested in medical questions. Did he nevertheless frequent doctors? On what terms was he with the younger Pinel, who was in charge of him in 1833? And with Dr. Fabre, his compatriot, whose Némésis médicale he illustrated? Who was the Dr. Court for whom he painted the water-color of les Médecins & la Mort *exhibited at the « Salon » of 1869? Why was he consulted when Rousseau's wife became mad and had to be put in the care of a doctor, and when Millet's wife had violent attacks of asthma? How can we explain the presence of* Diafoirus, *of* Imaginary Invalids, *of* Molière's Doctors *in the pictures painted about 1860? And, more generally, may not this taste for deforming his subjects have resulted from conversations with one of the disciples of Lavater?...*

The interest of the present collection is not confined, however, to showing what Daumier thought about doctors, as that prefaced by M. Julien Cain shows what he thought about the legal profession. These lithographs belong to different periods between 1833 and 1868 and thus allows us to appraise the successive styles of this great draftsman. First, we see the skillful lithographic draftsman, working for an audience that expected from him drawings they could recognize immediately and that would be always in the same style. At that time, he sought — and invariably found — his comic effects in the expressions of his subjects' faces. Robert Macaire, whom he portrayed and re-portrayed a hundred times, was exactly the type of thing people wanted from him and which he provided for his paper. He continued thus till about 1848, but from time to time he escaped from these conventional limits and revealed an artist much more remarkable and much more in advance of his time (the invalid in the Revue des peintres, *the housewife with a cold in the head, in* la Caricature provisoire). *The figures in the* Bons bourgeois, *specially the dentist (pl. 33) are already portrayed in a freer and more original way.*

In Paris grippé *(1858), we see a real change of style. The drawing has a range and acuteness that was lacking in the first period. For several years, Daumier's subjects* became mere pretexts, but at the same time we note the appearance of the theme of the doctor-wizard which links up with the Master's oil-paintings and water-colors.

This album reveals, moreover, the conditions under which the lithographer worked and his relationship with the Press, with his publishers and the Censorship. We have sought out the dates at which these works were executed — shown either by the number of the stone or by the date of deposit in the « Cabinet des Estampes » [Print Library] — because they are sometimes of interest. The plates were previously submitted to the Censorship and we note that they were generally sent in the form of proofs printed on one side of the paper, without any text on the back, fifteen days or a month before their publication in the journal to which Daumier contributed (the journal's own proofs carry the text on the back). However, one of the plates (Comment, docteur...) offers a more interesting field of research, for an examination of the above-mentioned elements reveal that it was lithographed in 1847, though it was not published till 1852.

This collection, which may appear arbitrary at first sight, thus opens the way, on the contrary, for far-reaching and as yet unattempted researches into the themes and art of our great Daumier.

JEAN ADHÉMAR

DESCRIPTIVE CATALOGUE

1. *Mr Prune.*   [*Mr. Prune.*]

June 26, 1833*. — Plate 288 of *la Caricature*, No. 138, June 27, 1833. — L. Delteil, No. 60 — Height : 259 × Width : 185**.

   Caricature of Dr. Prunelle (1777-1853), deputy, whose « bison's » head was a butt for jokes in the minor newspapers.

2. *Sage-femme. Mme de la Piçonnerie,...*   [*Midwife. — Mme de la Piçonnerie, sworn midwife, takes in paying guests for a just price.*]

July 7, 1833. — Plate 56 of the « Caricatures politiques » [Political Caricatures] published in *le Charivari*. — L. Delteil, No. 155. — H. 261 × W. 192.

   Field-Marshal Bugeaud had been entrusted with the mission of guarding the Duchesse de Berry in her prison at Blaye and supervising her confinement. This was the pretext for numerous jokes against him in the left-wing press, which named him « the midhusband ».

3. *Le Malade.*   [*The Sick Man.*]

June 5, 1835. — Plate 67, second stage published in the *Revue des Peintres*, 1835, vol. 14. — L. Delteil, No. 255, three stages described. — H. 183 × W. 142.

   A curious scene, surprising for its period, which is a distant forerunner of Millet's peasant subjects. The title may not be Daumier's. In any case, it is probable, in view of the review in which the scene was reproduced, that Daumier had used a subject of this sort in a painting and the review had asked him, according to its custom, to make a lithograph from it. Thus this may well be a copy made by the painter himself from one of his earliest pictures.

4. *La Potion.*   [*Medicine.*]

November 7, 1836. — « Galerie physionomique » [Studies in physiognomy], No. 2; published in *le Charivari* of November 19th 1836. — L. Delteil, No. 327. — H. 226 × W. 237.

   In this series (in which he collaborated with Traviès) Daumier concentrated on the expression on the faces of his models. The phial of copaiba indicates the disease from which the patient is suffering. — This series of lithographic prints appeared in *le Charivari* between November 1836 and December 1837.

5. *Vous mettrez aujourd'hui,...*   [*« Today, put in the column of Paris News : — The noted doctor Blaguefort (play on words : blague meaning a trick) has just succumbed to an attack of the disease that is now fashionable. This news has plunged the capital into deep sadness. — Tomorrow, you will insert a correction : — We have learned with pleasure that the noted Doctor Blaguefort has completely recovered*

---

 * Date of deposit of the duty copy.
 ** All dimensions are given in millimeters.

and resumed his consultations. — Every week put in a different little notice and come around each month for payment. »]

February 16, 1838. « Les Annonces » [News bulletins], No. 1, second stage published in *le Charivari* of March 13th 1838. — L. Delteil, No. 535, two stages described. — H. 213 × W. 206.

Daumier used this subject several times.
« Les Annonces », two plates published successively in *le Charivari* of March 13th and 18th, 1838.

6. *Robert Macaire philanthrope. — Vois-tu,...* [*Robert Macaire Philanthropist. — « You see, Bertrand, we are moralists in actions (play on words : actions also means stocks and bonds)... in actions that cost, naturally, 250 francs! We will treat the stockholders free of charge; you will purge them, I will bleed them. »*]

August 18, 1836. — « Caricaturana », No. 2, third stage published in *le Charivari* of August 28th 1836. — L. Delteil, No. 355, five stages described. — H. 272 × W. 227.

Charles Philipon, editor of *le Charivari*, asked Daumier for a series of lithographs on « Robert Macaire and Bertrand » and Gavarni for a series on « Robert Macaire as a Female » (which was later published under the title of *Fourberies de femmes en matière de sentiment* [How Women cheat at love]), so as to take advantage of the triumph of the great actor Frédérick Lemaître in Antier's play, *Robert Macaire*, which had been running for two years. Philipon composed the captions and claimed everywhere that he was himself the author of the series « Caricaturana », that was followed by a series of twenty more plates dealing with the same subject that appeared in the same review between October 1840 and September 1842. It is for this reason that some of the plates bear the words « Philipon invenit. H. Daumier lithogr. ».
In the second stage, the words *signerons* and *signerai* appeared in place of *soignerons* and *saignerai*, and *Beiftaeck* in place of *Beeftack*.

7. *Robert Macaire médecin. — Diable! ne plaisantez pas...* [*The Doctor Robert Macaire. — « For heaven's sake, don't take this sickness lightly!... Believe me, drink water, lots of water... rub the bones of your legs... and come to see me often... that won't impoverish you... my consultations are free... Now, you owe me 20 francs for these two bottles... (this includes 10 centimes deposit on each container). »*]

September 27, 1836. — « Caricaturana », No. 8, first stage (the second stage appeared in *le Charivari* of October 6th 1836). — L. Delteil, No. 361, three stages described. — H. 252 × W. 201.

This example — very rare according to Delteil — of a first printing, can be recognized by the caption : the words *On reprend le verre pour 10 centimes* are between brackets and are transcribed on the same line at the end of and following... *ces deux bouteilles,* whereas in the second (published) stage these words are placed a line further down and without brackets.

8. *Apothicaire et Pharmacien. — Mon cher Boniface,...* [*Apothecary and Druggist. — « My dear Boniface, it took an apothecary in the old days forty years to assure himself an annual income of 2.000 francs. You walked, we fly (volons : an untranslatable play on words, meaning both fly and steal). — But how do you manage? — We take some suet, crushed brick or starch, we call it Onicophane Ointment, or Racabout, or Nafé, or Osmaniglou, or any gibberish, then we advertise, send out prospectuses and circulars... and in 10 years we've made a million... We make a frontal attack on Fortune. You used to approach from the wrong side! »*]

May 25, 1837. — « Caricaturana », No. 53, second stage published in *le Charivari* of June 18th 1837. — L. Delteil, No. 408, three stages described. — H. 244 × W. 233.

It was this picture Flaubert had in mind when he created the character of M. Homais. The first rough drafts of *Madame Bovary* reveal this fact even more clearly than does the final text of the novel. In one of these rough drafts (Ms. g. 223², fol. 14, cf. éd. Gabrielle Leleu, I, p. 291) we read : « His house is plastered over with advertisements, those between the windows are in English script, in round-hand or print. « Vichy waters... Barèges, depurative treatment, Laffeteur, Darcet jujubes, Arab racahout, Nafé, « pectoral syrup, Regnault's lozenges,... » covers the whole length of the shop and bears in gold letters, with a dark border that makes them stand out in relief : *Homais, chemist.* Then, at the far end of the shop, above the copper scales fixed to the counter, one can see a door on which is written the word *Laboratory...* »

9. *Un oculiste breveté. — Ab! çà, Monsieur Macaire,...*   *[A Licensed Oculist. — «Listen, Mr. Macaire, for six montbs now you've been promising me wonders witb your marvelous eye-wasb, and still I'm blind. It ends up by costing me dear, my money is melting away, and tbat's all I see... — Well, at least tbat's sometbing; beep on, and you'll get to wbere you'll see clearly... (aside) in your pocbet boob.»]*
June 19, 1837. — «Caricaturana», No. 55, second stage published in *le Cbarivari* of July 2nd 1827. — L. Delteil, No. 410, two stages described. — H. 235 × W. 224.

10. *Robert Macaire dentiste. — Saprebleu! Mr le dentiste,...*   *[Robert Macaire, tbe Dentist. — «Great God, Doctor, you've pulled out two good teetb and left tbe two bad ones...» Dentist (aside) : «I'll be damned!... (Aloud) Of course I did, for good reasons. Tbere'll be plenty of time to pull out tbe bad ones... As for tbe otbers, tbey would eventually bave spoiled and caused you pain... A dental plate never burts, and it's rigbt in style. Everybody's wearing one.»]*
June 19, 1837. — «Caricaturana», No. 57, published in *le Cbarivari* of July 9th 1837. — L. Delteil, No. 412. — H. 232 × W. 218.

11. *Clinique du docteur Robert Macaire. — Hé bien! Messieurs,...*   *[Dr. Robert Macaire's Clinic. — «Tbere you are, gentlemen, you've seen tbis operation, tbat everyone said was impossible, performed witb complete success... — But, Doctor, tbe patient's dead... — Wbat of it! Sbe would bave died anyway even witbout tbe operation.»]*
August 30, 1837. — «Caricaturana», No. 63, published in *le Cbarivari* of October 15th 1837. — L. Delteil, No. 418. — H. 240 × W. 226.

12. *Tu vas porter cette note aux journaux.*   *[Tabe tbis release to tbe papers. — «A gentleman from tbe provinces after baving by mistabe swallowed a poucb (play on words : Avaler une blague means also to be taken in), and become suddenly bald and insolvent, tbe famous Doctor Robert Macaire concluded tbat poucbes (tricbs) wbicb ruin some, sbould, according to 'omiopatby' (for homeopathy), enricb otbers. Tbe treatment bas proved completely successful for bim. A bint to tbe wigs.» And, as I am named in tbis article, tomorrow, in accordance witb tbe law of tbe nintb of September 1835, I sball demand insertion of tbe following letter : «to tbe Editor,... I must request tbat you publisb in your paper tbe fact tbat I am not tbe source of tbe article, mentioning my name, tbat you publisbed yesterday. I do cure baldness (one, rue Belle Cbarge [Belle Charge means bigb fee]), but I treat it by a different metbod tban tbat you indicated. — Yours truly, Robert Macaire. 1, rue Belle Cbarge.»]*
October 30, 1837. — «Caricaturana», No. 66, second stage (the third stage was published in *le Cbarivari* of November 5th 1837). — L. Delteil, No. 421, three stages described. — H. 238 × W. 227.
    In this second stage, which is a rarity according to Delteil, *omiopatbique* replaces the word *boméopatbique* and we read *ce traitement lui a...* instead of *ce traitement médical lui a...* These errors necessitated the printing of a third stage. A compatriot and friend of Daumier, Dr. François Fabre (Fabre of Marseilles) pronounces a requisitory against homeopathy in his *Némésis médicale* (1840) illustrated by the Master :
        Disciples of Ahnemann, your misdeeds are known to us;
        We have made up our minds. Accuse us not of error;
        Your secrets have been revealed and in our tolerance
        We have carelessly allowed you to go too far.

13. *Fais bien attention! Si l'on te demande...*   *[«Listen carefully! If you're asbed for* muslim Rachout, *to fatten up all binds of sultanas, for* Arabian nafé *for sucbling cbildren of all ages, for* Oriental Kaiffa *to cure gastritis and corns, for* Teribronne *to stop vomiting, for* Amandine, Hindustani, Osman Igloo, Paraguay-Roux, Salep Chocolate, Hypocrasse, White Mustard *for blacb moods, tootb-acbe and deviations in beigbt, or* Giant Cabbage-seed, *you'll find it in tbis bag, tbe same one for tbem all, mabe no mistabe!!! and give it to 'em in tbe form of a powder, a paste, a solution or pellets, as you see fit. — Gee, wbat bind o' pellets are tbey, anyway? Tbey're fool pellets of tbe best quality. — Wonderful! Wonderful!»]*
November 15, 1837. — «Caricaturana», No. 69, first stage, previous to the various corrections made in the caption (the third stage was published in *le Cbarivari* of December 15th 1837). — L. Delteil, No. 424, three stages described. — H. 222 × W. 226.

14. *Le public, mon cher,...*   *[« The public, old fellow, is stupid... We bleed it, we physic it to death, and it's not satisfied... It wants a change... All right, let's give it something new, by becoming homœopaths... Similia similibus. » — Bertrand : « Amen ! » — « Look, here's a prescription that sums up the system : « Take a tiny grain of... nothing at all... separate it into 10 million molecules... throw one, « just one of these ten-millionth parts into the river... stir, until well mixed... let it steep several hours... fill « a pail with this healing water... filter... dilute with twenty parts of ordinary water... and wet the tongue « with it every morning before breakfast. » — Is that all ? — Yes... damn it, I forgot the most important part : « Pay for this prescription. »]*

November 21, 1837. — « Caricaturana », No. 70, first stage (the second stage was published in *le Charivari* of December 24th 1837). — L. Delteil, No. 425, two stages described. — H. 226 × W. 222.

    The second stage shows a change in the caption : after *homœopates* we read *il aime les blagues, traitons-le par des semblables*.

15. *Recette pour guérir la colique. — Mr Macaire,...*   *[How to cure the cramps. — « Mr. Macaire, my good friend, don't make me miss this performance, I need it badly. — Ah, my friend, I can't play, I'm in such pain... — Try, I beg you... the public is demanding you ; they're shouting, threatening, ready to rip out the seats. I'll have to return their money... Come, I'll double your bonus. — Oh, Oh, beat some towels... bring some hot wine, beat the towels. — I'll triple your bonus. — Keep the beat on... keep beating the towels. — We'll share the box office receipts. — We'll share the box office receipts ? Up with the curtain. The farce is ended, the drama begins... »]*

January 11, 1838. — « Caricaturana », No. 72, second stage published in *le Charivari* of January 14th 1838. — L. Delteil, No. 427, three stages described. — H. 233 × W. 231.

    In the third stage the No. 72, top right, is placed obliquely.

16. *Le début. — (Bertrand) Oh ! non, la malade,...*   *[The Beginners. — Bertrand : « Oh no, the patient is weak, she wouldn't survive : the operation is impracticable... » Robert Macaire : « Impracticable ! ! ! Nothing is impracticable for a beginner. Listen, we have no name yet among the profession. If we fail, we don't lose anything. If, by chance we succeed... well, we'll be launched, our reputation will be made. » Both : « Let's go ahead then. »]*

January 30, 1838. — « Caricaturana », No. 75, second stage published in *le Charivari* of March 6th 1838. — L. Delteil, No. 430, two stages described. — H. 248 × W. 225.

17. *Robert Macaire magnétiseur. — Voici un excellent sujet...*   *[Robert Macaire, the hypnotizer. — « Here is an excellent subject for hypnotism. There is absolutely no connivance ; I don't even know Mademoiselle de St. Bertrand, and you are going to see, gentlemen, the effect of somnambulism... » — (Mlle. de St. Bertrand gives, in her sleep, consultations on one's illnesses, tells where treasures are hidden in the ground, advises buying stock in the Mozart Paper Co., in gold mines, or in a number of other fine enterprises.)]*

July 21, 1838. — « Caricaturana », No. 88, second stage published in *le Charivari* of August 26th 1838. — L. Delteil, No. 443, two stages described. — H. 236 × W. 234.

    At this period, Balzac, like Daumier, was greatly interested in hypnotism (see *Ursulé Mirouet*, published in 1841, and *La Dernière Incarnation de Vautrin*, 1846). The previous year in 1837, the Academy of Medicine had carried out an enquiry on the subject of hypnotism after a young hypnotist named Berna had submitted his discoveries to it (A. Binet and Ch. Féré, *Le Magnétisme animal*, p. 29). The triumph of hypnotism did not occur till about 1840 (cf. works by Dr. Alphonse Teste and especially his *Manuel pratique de magnétisme animal*, 1840 ; l'*Histoire académique du magnétisme animal*, by Cl. Burdin, 1841 ; the second edition, 1840, of the *Cours* by Baron J. du Potel de Sennery, future publisher of the *Journal du Magnétisme*).

18. *B'en parlez pas, j' suis enrubé...*   *[« Don't talk, I bab such a co'd in by head that I can't see straight, by dear !... »]*

April 20, 1839. — First stage published in *la Caricature provisoire* No. 25 of April 21st 1839. — L. Delteil, No. 560, two stages described. — H. 220 × W. 275.

Here we have one of the first examples of Daumier's new style of caricature, in which he suddenly began to concentrate on faces and expressions instead of on the whole attitude, as hitherto. A cold in the head serves him as a fine excuse for showing the contrasting profiles of these two women.

The first stage appeared in *La Caricature provisoire*, a non-political journal founded by Philipon in order to earn money to pay the fines inflicted on the ferocious *Caricature*. The second stage appeared on September 5th, 1841 in *le Charivari*.

19. *Une envie de femme grosse.*   *[Cravings of a pregnant woman.]*

« Mœurs conjugales » [Married Life], No. 15, second stage published in *le Charivari* of November 2-3, 1839. — L. Delteil, No. 638, two stages described. — H. 234 × W. 199.

20. *Monsieur est malade,...*   *[« The Master is ill and will receive nobody ».]*

September 27, 1839. — « Émotions parisiennes » [Parisian events], second stage (the third stage appeared in *le Charivari* of October 6th 1839). — L. Delteil, No. 690, three stages described. — H. 240 × W. 177.

In the second stage, the comma between the words *malade* and *il* is omitted.

21. *Le Médecin et la garde-malade.*   *[The Doctor and the Nurse. — « How is the patient ? — Alas, he died this morning at 6 o'clock. — Ah, then he didn't take my medicine. — But he did, sir. — Then he must have taken too much. — No, Doctor. — Then, he didn't take enough of it. »]*

June 27, 1840. — « Émotions parisiennes » [Parisian events], No. 30, second stage (the third stage appeared in *le Charivari* of July 6th 1840). — L. Delteil, No. 714, three stages described. — H. 223 × W. 188.

This dialogue between a doctor and a nurse precedes by six years that between Madame Cibot and Dr. Poulain in Balzac's *Le Cousin Pons* : « Sensitive, devoted Cibot fetched the local doctor. In Paris, there exists in each quarter a doctor whose name and address are known only to the people of the working class, to small bourgeois and janitors, and who is known as the local doctor...

The words *il est mort, le gaillard*, following the *Ah!...* do not appear in the second stage, in which Aubert's address is given in the middle.

22. *Elle tenait ferme!...*   *[It certainly was solid!]*

August 8, 1839. — « Scènes grotesques » [Grotesque scenes], No. 4, second stage published in *le Charivari* of August 10th 1839. — L. Delteil, No. 732, two stages described. — H. 202 × W. 190.

« Scènes grotesques » (a series of six plates published in *le Charivari* between June 19th and November 29th, 1839). The grotesque quality of theses scenes is partly due to the fact that the characters have small bodies and huge heads. André Gill was later to make use of and develop the same comic convention.

23. *La Garde-malade. — Décidément,...*   *[The Nurse. — « No doubt about it, fruit venders are the only ones who introduce you to interesting people. An epilectic, a hydrophobic and a lunatic!... And in addition, if the grocer can get me that tuberculosis he promised me, that would be darned nice for me. »]*

December 26, 1841. — « Bohémiens de Paris » [Parisian bohemians], No. 15, second stage published in *la Caricature*, 3rd year (the fifth stage appeared in *le Charivari* of May 22nd 1842). — L. Delteil, No. 836, five stage described. — H. 245 × W. 178.

This plate was published four times : according to the different captions, it portrayed a janitress, then an old street-walker, before it came to represent a nurse. There exists a painting on this subject which is attributed to Daumier.

24. *Le Malade imaginaire. — Cette classe de citoyens...* [*The Hypochondriac. — This category of citizen is the providence of the medical profession, the benediction of the drug trade. It is the nymph Egeria whose inspiration was responsible for white mustard, red Paraguay, Regnault paste, the Clyso-bol, and in general all inventions for relieving unsuffering humanity. The hypochondriac is the prey, one after the other of pleurisy, consumption and so forth and so forth... He varies his ills in order to vary his pleasures and every day he exclaims when he feels his pulse : «Really, my health must be good and sound to be able to resist all these diseases.»*]

December 1840. — «Monomanes» [Monomaniacs], No. 7, first stage, with the addition of an incomplete manuscript letter (the second stage appeared in *le Charivari* of January 18th 1841). — L. Delteil, No. 864, two stages described. — H. 218 × W. 193.

«Les Monomanes» (a series of eight plates published in *le Charivari*, pl. 1, 2 and 4-8; and in *la Caricature*, pl. 3, from 1840 to 1841) portray, as well as the imaginary invalid : le *bétophile* (canary-lover), the embroiderer, the scholar, the amateur guitarist, the regulator, the Parisian page-boy. The manuscript caption on this proof does not seem to have been written by Daumier as are several of those preserved in the same collection (Dc 180 c Rés.).

25. *Le strabisme, ma foi,...* [*The Squint. — «Lord! I didn't recognize you! — Oh, that's because I had an operation. I'm no longer cross-eyed, and that changes my looks completely, don't you think so? — Yes, completely. Before, you squinted toward the outside...»*]

April 1841. — «Actualités» [Current events], No. 48, second stage published in *la Caricature* of April 11th 1841. — L. Delteil, No. 916, two stages described. — H. 225 × W. 227.

In the second stage, «No. 48» appears on the top right.

26. *Le Médecin hydropathe. — Aujourd'hui...* [*The Hydropathic Doctor. — «Today, two bucketsful will do... tomorrow you can bring four. — Ah, what a fine doctor!... One can't like water too much... (aside) I'm only afraid it'll end up by killing his taste for food forever!...»*]

October 1842. — «Caricatures du jour» [Present day caricatures], No. 50, second stage published in *la Caricature* of October 30th 1842. — L. Delteil, No. 995, three stages described. — H. 189 × W. 223.

This kind of treatment was still a novelty. In his novel, *Jérôme Paturot*, 1843, Louis Reybaud shows us, as did Daumier, «*les hydropathes*, a new invention, school of the German Priessnitz... No more cures except by pure water... — This, Saint-Ernest, is as yet little known...». — The second stage does not show the title of the series : «Caricatures du jour».

27. *Une heureuse trouvaille. — Parbleu...* [*A Lucky Find. — «By Jove, I'm delighted! You have yellow fever... it will be the first time I've been lucky enough to treat this disease!»*]

September 1844. — «Les Beaux jours de la vie» [Red letter days], No. 23, second stage (the third stage appeared in *le Charivari* of September 11th 1844). — L. Delteil, No. 1110, three stages described. — H. 220 × W. 220.

A third stage had to be printed after the above, because the author of the caption insisted that the word *Parbleu* must be followed by an exclamation mark, which does not appear here. This detail proves the interest taken by the public in the captions, to which, we are told, they paid more attention than to the pictures.

28. *Les Cigarettes de camphre. — On m'a certifié...* [*Camphor cigarettes. — «I've been told they're wonderful for putting on weight!... — And I've been assured that they're infallible for reducing!...»*]

December 1845. — «Les Beaux jours de la vie» [Red letter days], No. 81, second stage published in *le Charivari* of January 4th 1846. — L. Delteil, No. 1169, two stages described. — H. 234 × W. 231.

In the figure on the right, Daumier made use of a type resembling Balzac, recognizable by the long hair, hat, fleshy face and stoutness. The great caricaturist had what Mr. Roberts-Jones has called his

« familiar passers-by », who were the persons, friends or men encountered in the street, whom he depicted in his various physiognomic portrait galleries.

« Les Beaux jours de la vie » comprises a hundred plates, many of them excellent, published in *le Charivari* between December 24th 1843 and September 19th 1846.

29. *Vois-tu cet imbécile...* [*« Look at this fool who does not even notice that his barrell is leaking... — You're ignorant! It is on purpose, it's chloride which is being sprayed on the streets to disinfect them... it's the Labaraque system, applied to the city of Paris. »*]

August 1844. — « Les Étrangers à Paris » [Foreigners in Paris], No. 19, second stage published in *le Charivari* of August 28th 1844. — L. Delteil, No. 1290, two stages described. — H. 229 × W. 181.

An allusion to the chemist Antoine Labarraque (1777-1850), who carried out research on the subject of disinfection and who was awarded the Montyon Prize for his discovery of the importance of potassium-chloride water in this sphere.

30. *Hier, dans la rue Saint-Honoré,...* [*Yesterday in the Rue Saint-Honoré, a dignified elderly man was felled by an attack of apoplexy. It would have been the end of him if by chance the well known Dr. Cabassol who happened to be at his window at No. 107, had not hastened to his help. Thanks to his intelligent treatment and devoted care, the patient was quickly revived. Our famous Dr. Cabassol, adding to his generous attentions, refused to accept any payment other than the thanks of a family that will eternally bless his name. Glory to Dr. Cabassol. — « You know, you're the one who was the dignified old man. You might have fallen on your way to see me yesterday, you might have hurt yourself, and then I could have come to your help. I have presented all this in a more dramatic way for the newspapers. It won't do you any harm and it'll do me a lot of good!... »*]

October 1844. — « Les Philanthropes du jour » [The present day philanthropists], No. 9, second stage published in *le Charivari* of October 26th 1844. — L. Delteil, No. 1300, two stages described. — H. 233 × W. 181.

31. *Oui monsieur...* [*« Yes sir... dedicated by my profession and my sentiments to the purest philanthropy, I have not hesitated to spend my nights nor to use up my retorts and stills, to discover a salve more Regnauld (Regnauld was the name of a popular salve) than anything known to this day... I have finally realized my dreams... that is to say, the fusion of wood lice and slugs... as my first care is to relieve suffering and coughing humanity, in spite of the high price of the raw materials, I sell the box for only five francs... half a box cured Mr. Ducantal senior... »*]

November 1844. — « Les Philanthropes du jour » [The present day philanthropists], No. 18, second stage published in *le Charivari* of November 18th 1844. — L. Delteil, No. 1310, two stages described. — H. 229 × W. 180.

An allusion to Regnault's lozenges from which Dr. Véron had made his fortune. This Véron was frequently a target for jokes in *le Charivari*, where he was considered as the symbol of the pot-bellied, opportunistic bourgeois. Regnault, a chemist in the rue Caumartin, had never managed to persuade the public to buy his cough lozenges. They were launched by Dr. Véron after his death.

32. *Mon cher, je t'assure...* [*« My dear fellow, I give you my word that you look very ill this morning. I'm talking not as your doctor but as your friend, I insist on treating you... better than I would myself. I'm going to apply thirty leeches to your epigastrium and if tomorrow I don't find you improved, I'll apply sixty... »*]

August 1845. — « Les Amis » [The friends], No. 8, second stage published in *le Charivari* of August 18th 1845. — L. Delteil, No. 1386, two stages described. — H. 235 × W. 185.

The last of a series of nine plates on the subject of « Friends », published in *le Charivari* of May 9th-August 23rd 1845.

33. *Ob! là... là... là... là!... — Tant mieux...* [*«Oucb!... Oucb!... — Fine... fine... that proves it's coming!...»*]

November 1846. — « Les Bons bourgeois » [The good bourgeois], No. 45, second stage published in *le Charivari* of May 4th 1847. — L. Delteil, No. 1521, two stages described. — H. 249 × W. 212.

The date of deposit here precedes that of publication by seven months. Here, Daumier's style is no longer that of 1845, or rather, he had managed to persuade his editor to publish a drawing in a less traditional style.

« Les Bons bourgeois » comprises the famous series of eighty-two plates published in *le Charivari* between May 1st 1846 and June 1849.

34. *Ab! docteur...* [*«Doctor, I believe I'm consumptive.»*]

July 1847. — « Tout ce qu'on voudra » [Anything you like], No. 18, second stage published in *le Charivari* of October 19th 1847. — L. Delteil, No. 1664, two stages described. — H. 248 × W. 216.

In order to satisfy his publisher, Daumier was forced to use the same theme several times. Here we see a subject he had already treated in 1845 (pl. 32). The number of the lithographic stone (1024) proves that it does indeed date from 1847 and that Daumier had lithographed two hundred plates since the example from the series entitled « Les Amis », which is described above.

« Tout ce qu'on voudra » is a series of seventy numbered plates published in *le Charivari* between March 28th 1847 and July 19th 1851.

35. *Le Malade : comment, docteur,...* [*«The patient : «What, doctor! Not even a soft boiled egg!» — The doctor : «No, you'll have to keep to the strictest diet for five more days... It's a mistake to think we must eat to live!... Excuse me if I run along, I have a dinner engagement!...»*]

June 1852. — « Tout ce qu'on voudra » [Anything you like], an unnumbered series, second stage published in *le Charivari* of June 19th 1852. — L. Delteil, No. 2204, two stages described. — H. 244 × W. 216.

The print shows the stone number 1007, which signifies that it dates from 1847 and, like many of Daumier's stones, was not used till 1852. There is something symptomatic about the title « Tout ce qu'on voudra », bestowed on these eighteen stones that had already grown old.

36. *Le Docteur Véron ayant renoncé...* [*Doctor Véron having renounced politics, its pomp and its works, retires to the country, at Auteuil and devotes himself to the favorite pastimes of the Arcadian shepherds of old; the true sage consoles himself with some philosophy and clarinet.*]

« Actualités » [Current events], second stage published in *le Charivari* of June 25th 1852. — L. Delteil, No. 2257, two stages described. — H. 257 × W. 220.

Dr. Véron, a remarkable business man, had earned a considerable fortune, first by launching pectoral lozenges, then by founding a newspaper. Thiers entrusted him with the direction of the Opera-house in Paris, then dismissed him after a few years, accusing him (according to Véron himself) of having succeeded, and earned large sums for the State. After this incident he retired to his house in Auteuil.

37. *Paris grippé. — Comment toussez-vous?...* [*The Grippe Epidemic in Paris. — «How are you coughing? — I'm coughing quite well, thank you,... and you?»*]

January 30, 1858. — « Croquis parisiens » [Parisian sketches], 8th series, No. 43, second stage published in *le Charivari* of February 1st 1858. — L. Delteil, No. 3022, two stages described. — H. 208 × W. 251.

There had been several epidemics of influenza in France, one in 1837, the others in 1842 and 1847, the latter not being severe. Early in 1858, however, an extremely bad epidemic broke out, following, according to Dr. Ph. Bernard « specially prolonged and serious attacks of typhoid » (*Étude chronologique de certaines épidémies...*, 1935). The same author observes that, from 1860 on, « there has been a slight, uninterrupted little epidemic each year ».

38. *Viens donc..., mon ami,...*   [*«Come along, dear, I don't think that picture pretty. — Oh! yes, it is... as a pharmacist it interests me greatly. The picture certainly represents the testing of a new medicine... let's see what the catalogue says?...»*]

June 3, 1859. — «Exposition de 1859» [The exhibition of 1859], No. 11, second stage published in *le Charivari* of June 21st 1859. — L. Delteil, No. 3143, two stages described. — H. 211 × W. 265.

It is possible, though it cannot be affirmed because of the lack of any known reproduction, that this is a caricature of *l'Amour piqué* by Jules-Eugène Lenepveu (No. 1940 in the 1859 «Salon»).

«L'Exposition de 1859» (a series of nine irregularly numbered plates published in *le Charivari* from April 6th to June 21st 1859). — Stone No. 37.

39. *Esculape se mettant en garde...*   [*Esculapius, prepared to defend energetically his position against all innovators (blond or dark), who come to attack it.*]

March 16, 1859. — «Actualités» [Current events], No. 20, second stage published in *le Charivari* of March 29th 1859. — L. Delteil, No. 3133, two stages described. — H. 226 × W. 264.

In 1859, a certain Vriès, known as the Black Doctor (hence Daumier's allusion to Blacks and Whites), who claimed to be able to cure cancer, was condemned by the Academy of Medicine following a report by Dr. Velpeau.

40. *Paris grippé.*   [*Paris in the throes of the grippe.*]

February 13, 1864. — «Actualités» [Current events], No. 33, second stage published in *le Charivari* of February 18th 1864. — L. Delteil, No. 3269, two stages described. — H. 242 × W. 220.

41. *Voyons... ouvrons la bouche!...*   [*«Come on... let's open our mouth.»*]

February 17, 1864. — «Les Moments difficiles de la vie» [The hard moments in life], No. 1, second stage published in *le Charivari* of March 12th 1864. — L. Delteil, No. 3272, two stages described. — H. 241 × W. 204.

One of a series in which Daumier experimented in the depiction of figures with their heads thrown back; the figure of the dentist and the story in the picture were secondary considerations.

«Les Moments difficiles de la vie» (a series of seven plates numbered 1-6 [the seventh having been rejected] published in *le Charivari* from March 12th to July 6th, 1864).

42. *Vous ne prenez rien?...*   [*«Aren't you taking anything? — No, I'm afraid. — Oh, come! a laudanum grog!»*]

October 24, 1865. — «Croquis parisiens» [Parisian sketches], No. 16, second stage published in *le Charivari* of November 2-3rd 1865. — L. Delteil, No. 3434, two stages described. — H. 245 × W. 228.

Daumier had left the Ile Saint-Louis for Montmartre and chiefly frequented a café in the Place Pigalle. He was depicting scenes in cafés and saloons. Since the public took no interest in this type of scene, he made no paintings of them, whereas a little later Manet and Degas, who had followed his work, painted *l'Absinthe* and *Au Café*.

43. *Hier le fusil à aiguille,...*   [*«Yesterday the breech-loading gun (aiguille refers to steel igniting pin of such a gun), tomorrow, those fellows. Will we be better off?»*]

May 28, 1867. — «Actualités» [Current events], No. 104, second stage published in *le Charivari* of June 8th 1867. — L. Delteil, No. 3577, two stages described. — H. 259 × W. 223.

Congress held during the year of the Universal Exhibition, coinciding with the arrival of the King and Crown Prince of Prussia and the Emperor of Russia. Here, Daumier recalls the threat to France constituted by the armament of Prussia, after her victory at Sadowa. This *International Congress of Medicine*, the first of its kind, actually took place at the end of August. The discussions chiefly concerned measures against the propagation of venereal disease.

44. *Réception académique.*   [*Academic Reception.*]

April 17, 1868. « Actualités » [Current events], No. 97, second stage (the third stage appeared in *le Charivari* of April 24th 1868). — L. Delteil, No. 3636, three stages described. — H. 244 × W. 224.

The reception was that of Jules Favre, successor to Victor Cousin, elected on May 2nd 1868 and admitted the following year by Charles de Rémusat.

The second stage still shows an « error » : *reception* in place of *réception.*

45. *La colique. — Holà! Holà!...*   [*Cramps. — « Oh! Oh! Oh! my stomach! »*]

« L'Imagination » [Imagination], No. 6, second stage published in *le Charivari* of February 19th 1833. — L. Delteil, app. No. 34, two stages described. — H. 238 × W. 200.

This plate belongs to the series « l'Imagination » (fifteen plates) composed by Daumier in prison, where he had been detained since August 31st 1832 for « inciting to hatred and contempt of the Government ». The series, published in *le Charivari* from January 14th to October 19th 1833, was signed by Charles Ramelet, an obscure professional lithographer, who was a friend and imitator of the Master. However, Ramelet may have been merely a figure-head. It should be noted that Daumier was not interned at that time at Sainte-Pélagie, but in the house of Dr. J.-P.-Casimir Pinel, nephew of the specialist in mental diseases, to whom men condemned for offenses in the Press were sent after spending a certain time in prison. This system, of assimilating opposition journalists to mental patients, has received insufficient attention.

46. *Le Mal de tête. — Holà! holà!...*   [*The Headache. — « Oh! Oh! Bang-bang-ding-a-ling Oh! »*]

« L'Imagination » [Imagination], No. 9, second stage published in *le Charivari* of April 23rd 1833. — L. Delteil, app. No. 37, two stages described. — H. 235 × W. 195.

It is possible that this series, composed and no doubt lithographed by Daumier when he was staying with Dr. Pinel, was inspired by the latter.

Pinel, the nephew, born at Saint-Paul (Tarn) in 1800, was in charge of a clinic for nervous and mental diseases at Chaillot (79, Champs-Elysées) which he later transferred to la Folie-Saint-James. He had been an Army surgeon and was given his diploma as a doctor in 1826. Like his cousin Scipion and his relative Eugène, he was the author of works on mental illness (1856).

The little demons were indispensable to the imagery of the period. Gavarni published several series on this theme from 1824, but they were a speciality of Ernest Lepoitevin (1806-1870) whose two albums entitled *Les diables de lithographies* were published by Aumont and by Tilt.

47. *Le Malade imaginaire. — Je suis perdu...*   [*The Hypochondriac. — « I'm done for... I'll have to make my will... They're going to bury me... farewell. »*]

« L'Imagination » [Imagination], No. 10, second stage published in *le Charivari* of May 21st 1833. — L. Delteil, app. No. 38, two stages described. — H. 240 × W. 190.

48. *Le Médecin. — Pourquoi, diable!...*   [*The Doctor. — « How the devil does it happen that all my patients succumb?... Yet I bleed them, I physic them, I drug them... I simply can't understand! »*]

« L'Imagination » [Imagination], No. 15, second stage published in *le Charivari* of August 19th 1833. — L. Delteil, app. No. 43, two stages described. — H. 249 × W. 199.